A QUIET RETURN
TO WHAT THE
BODY ONCE KNEW

THE RHYTHM
OF HEALTH

KERRY KING

The Rhythm of Health

Copyright © 2025 Kerry King

All rights reserved. No part of this book may be reproduced, stored in a retrieval system, or transmitted in any form or by any means, electronic, mechanical, photocopying, recording, or otherwise, without prior written permission from the copyright holder, except brief quotations used in reviews or critical articles.

ISBN 978 1 7642659 0 4 (Paperback)
ISBN 978 1 7642659 1 1 (Hardback)
ISBN 978 1 7642659 2 8 (Audiobook)
ISBN 978 1 7642659 3 5 (eBook)

First Edition

Cover image: Adobe Stock

Typeset in Cormorant Garamond by Christian Thalmann and Montserrat by Julieta Ulanovsky

Printed and bound in Australia

A catalogue record for this book is available from the National Library of Australia

Disclaimer: This book is intended for general information purposes only. It is not a substitute for medical advice, diagnosis, or treatment. Readers should consult a qualified health professional before making any changes to diet, lifestyle, or healthcare.

There was a time when health was not a puzzle.
It was the rhythm of waking with the light,
moving with the day,
and resting with the night.

This book is a quiet return,
not to something new,
but to what the body has always known.

A Message from the Author

I didn't write this because I had all the answers. I wrote this because I didn't. For years, I struggled. Pain. Exhaustion. Frustration. I read the books, tried the plans, followed the advice, and still felt like something was missing.

This book came from the search to find what actually works. Not just for health. But for balance. For rhythm. For peace. It isn't filled with studies or academic references. It's the fruit of years of living, testing, and learning what truly restores health.

Health has been made too complicated. Layered with jargon, hype, and endless rules. But it was never meant to be that way. This book is simple on purpose. It will guide you slowly and gently through the rhythms that restore.

I'm someone who has walked through the fog and found my way out. This is the map I wish I had. So, if you've been trying everything and still feel stuck, here is your map home.

You're not broken. You're just out of rhythm.
And rhythm can be restored.

Kerry King

Important Note Before You Begin

This guide was written to support you, not to diagnose, treat, or cure any condition. It offers insight drawn from lived experience, clinical observation as an Osteopath, and study, but it's not a substitute for professional medical advice. Think of this as a companion to your current care, not a replacement.

Not every section in this book will be right for every person, and that's okay. If you're unsure, take it to your doctor or healthcare provider - especially if you're pregnant, breastfeeding, managing a health condition, or taking prescription medication. They may tell you that certain practices don't suit your body right now. That doesn't mean the rest won't help. Begin with the pieces that fit. As your body heals, more may become possible later. Even small steps can restore rhythm.

As your health shifts, you may notice changes in energy, digestion, or blood markers, and your medication needs may change with them. If you take prescriptions for things like blood pressure, thyroid, or cholesterol, make changes slowly and with support.

Use what resonates, and take responsibility for your own choices. The author and publisher aren't liable for any outcomes that may result from how you use the information in these pages.

Ask questions. Go gently. You're not alone.

Table of Contents

Introduction: What is Health? — 1

The Body's Circuit — 5
  Reception — 9
  Transmission — 11
  Regulation — 13
  Conversion — 17
  Expression — 20
  Protection — 22
  Reset — 26

The Seven Pillars of Health — 35

The Six-Phase Reset — 61

Phase 1: Build the Foundation — 67
  Breathe Deep — 68
  Light that Charges — 71
  First Hydrate — 75
  Let Movement Flow — 81

Phase 2: Reset the Body Clock — 87
  Let Light In — 88
  Eat in Time — 91
  Return to Dark — 94
  Sleep Deep — 98

Phase 3: The Right Environment — 107
  Clean the Air — 108
  Honour the Surface — 111
  Make Room to Breathe — 114
  Ground the Body — 117
  Restore the Gut — 120

Phase 4: Build Your Mitochondria — 127
    Embrace the Cold — 128
    Build Strength — 132
    Restorative Light — 136

Phase 5: Fuel the Fire — 143
    Return to Ancestral Fuel — 146
    Opening the Pantry — 147
    Not All Meat is the Same — 148
    What About Plants? — 151
    Let's Talk about Fats and Oils — 156
    What You Drink Matters — 160
    How to Cook, Store and Prepare Food — 164
    Choosing Your Starting Point — 168
    Build Meals That Burn Clean — 172
    The Reintroduction Roadmap — 177

Phase 6: Live in Rhythm — 185
    Work in Rhythm — 187
    Rest in Rhythm — 190
    Play in Rhythm — 193
    Walk the Seasons — 196

The Final Word — 205

Appendix — 211
    Reference Map — 212
    Rhythm Summary — 213
    The Return Path — 216
    When You've Tried Everything — 218
    Troubleshooting & FAQs — 220
    Oxalate Dumping — 225
    Choosing a Red Light Device — 226
    Bone Broth Recipe — 227
    If You Want to Go Deeper — 228

Introduction
What is Health?

What is Health, Really?

What if health wasn't something you had to chase? What if it wasn't a list of rules, or rigid plans? What if your body already knew what to do, and just needed the right conditions to remember?

This book isn't here to make you feel like you're behind, broken, or not doing enough. It's here as an invitation to return. To the rhythm your body was always designed to follow.

Health isn't just what you do, it's when you do it. When you move in time with it, things begin to shift. Energy flows clearer. Sleep deepens. Hunger balances. Mood steadies. Stress softens. It's not magic. It's timing.

This rhythm runs *daily* - through light and dark. It runs *weekly* - in cycles of movement and rest. And it runs *seasonally* - as your body responds to the world around it.

You've likely felt this before, even without words for it. That calm after an early walk. That deep sleep in the cool, dark. That focus after time away from screens. That's not just preference, that's design. This book will help you return to that design.

So Where Do You Begin?

You begin with flow. Your body runs on an internal circuit that receives light, moves charge, makes energy and expresses through movement, thought and speech. This circuit is always running, even when you can't feel it. When it's blocked or overwhelmed, your whole system suffers.

That flow of energy depends on what you take in day to day. The air you breathe, the light around you, the way you fuel and hydrate. All of it feeds into the circuit. Each input plays a different role in keeping energy moving. Together, they shape your health. How well you recover. How easily your body finds balance.

This book will guide you through both - how your body flows, and what it needs to keep that flow steady. Not through strict plans or pressure, but through the rhythms and fuels your body remembers. And finally, step by step, you'll be led through a Six-Phase Reset, one rhythm at a time, back towards the pattern your body was always designed to follow.

How to Read This Book

The next couple of chapters go a bit deeper into how the body works and what fuels the system. They matter, they're the foundation, but they can feel heavier than what follows.

If you find yourself slowing down or feeling weighted by detail, that's okay. You can move ahead to the practical Six-Phase Reset chapters and let them breathe first. You can always circle back to the earlier chapters later when you're ready.

This isn't a book you read once and put away. It's a map. And with a map, you don't try to memorise every turn, you keep coming back to it. You'll flick forward, you'll flick back, you'll reread sections, sometimes five times. That's how it's meant to be read.

So move through the map at your own pace, and in your own way. Listen to your body. Let it guide you.

The Body as a Circuit
Seven Layers of Electrical Flow

The Body as a Circuit

What if Your Body Is a Living Circuit, Not a Machine?

You're not just a mix of organs and systems doing their own thing. Your body is *electric*. Every single process, every heartbeat, every breath, every thought runs on charge. And that charge doesn't move randomly. It flows through a circuit. Just like a house needs wiring to carry light, your body needs structure to carry charge. And just like circuits can short out, your body can too when the signals get blocked, the wires are jammed, or the flow can't return. Your health depends on how well this circuit moves.

This isn't something you feel with sparks or shocks. But it is there, underneath everything. When it flows well, you feel clear, calm, steady. When it doesn't, energy slows, and your body starts working harder than it should.

The Seven Layers of Electrical Flow

1. Reception | The Solar Panels

Your body absorbs light and signal from the world around you. This is where the circuit begins, if you don't receive well, there's no energy to flow.

2. Transmission | The Wires

Once light energy is received, it moves through your water, blood and lymph. These are your body's liquid wires carrying charge.

3. Regulation | The Insulation

The encasing of every cell acts as insulation. They control what stays in, what stays out, and govern how energy is regulated.

4. Conversion | The Engine

Mitochondria are the engines of our cells. They take fat and oxygen - and with the help of light - make ATP, the fuel your body runs on.

5. Expression | The Output Channels

Energy from ATP is used outwardly for movement, thought, and speech. And inwardly to make hormones, repair, and heal.

6. Protection | The Shield

Fascia and your body's electromagnetic field (biofield) guard the system. They protect the circuit and help you stay calm, clear, and stable. If those words feel new, don't worry, they'll be explained later.

7. Reset | The Return Path

Every system needs a release. Through rest, detox, and elimination, your body resets and finds balance again.

This is the structure your body was built on. It's a living circuit. When one link breaks the whole circuit trips. But when the current flows unbroken, the body can begin to heal.

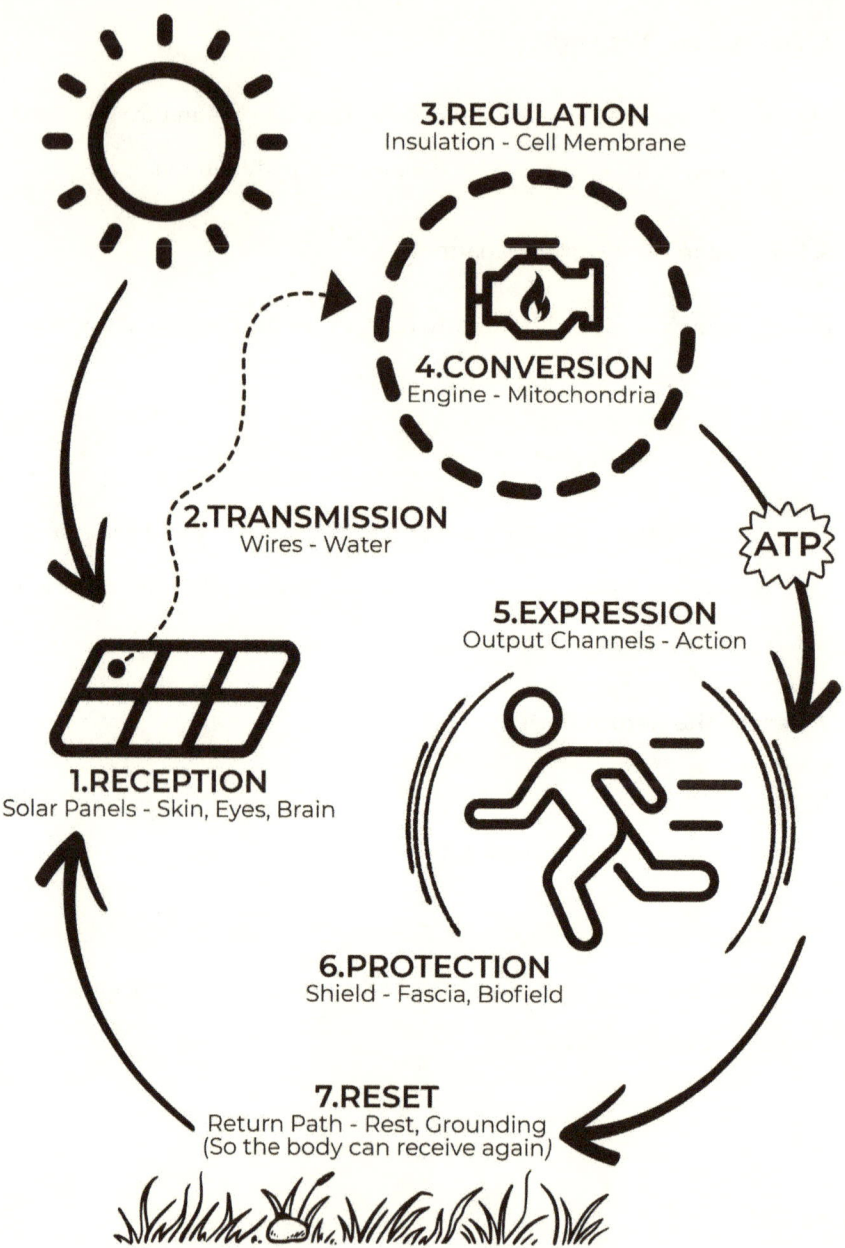

Picture: The Body as a Circuit | Above is a simple sketch of your circuit. Let the arrows show the path. If you lose your place in the chapters, come back to this page.

1. Reception | The Solar Panels

Reception is the first layer of your body's circuit. And it begins with light. Melanin, the pigment in your skin, works like solar panels - catching sunlight and turning it into charge that flows into your body's wires. This is the spark. When reception is clear, every layer downstream has a chance to run in rhythm. Miss the signal, and the circuit grows dim.

The Disconnect

Too much indoor light. Too much screen time. Routines that disconnect you from the sun. The body stops catching real signals and starts chasing artificial ones.

You feel flat in the mornings, even after sleep. Your skin looks dull. You reach for coffee. You feel cut off from nature, time, and even yourself. You forget what it feels like to burn from the inside.

How It Can Show Up

When light is missed, the spark is lost. The following conditions show how broken reception can appear in the body. They're here to help you see the thread beneath, not to diagnose.

- Fatigue
- Seasonal Affective Disorder
- Vitamin D Deficiency
- Depression or Low Mood
- Slow Recovery from Illness
- Weak Immunity

When It's Flowing

You wake with ease. Your skin looks alive, not drained. Your body feels charged just from standing in sunlight. You feel connected to your surroundings, not foggy, not distant. There's a quiet hum under your skin, like your body is pulsing with life.

2. Transmission | The Wires

Once energy is received, it has to move. That's the job of your fluid wires - your blood, lymph, and water. These are the body's inner rivers. Every beat, every breath, sends charge through. Without flow, the body becomes tired, stuck, and dry.

The Disconnect

Dehydration stalls transmission. But dehydration isn't only about not drinking enough, it's also when the body's fluids become stagnant. Long periods of sitting, low-quality water, poor circulation, can all leave the body "dry on the inside" even if you're drinking all day. The wires start to fray. The current slows.

You feel cloudy. You get dizzy when standing. Your skin looks tight or dull. Constipation, cold fingers, brain fog, or sudden drops in energy show up. You drink more but never feel fully hydrated, like your body just isn't absorbing what you give it.

How It Can Show Up

When water doesn't carry charge well, flow stalls. The following conditions show how broken transmission can appear in the body.

- Headaches
- Dizziness and POTS
- Muscle Cramps
- Restless Leg Syndrome
- Dry Skin, Eyes, Mouth
- Poor Cold Tolerance
- Poor Heat Tolerance
- Fatigue and Brain Fog
- Kidney Stones
- Constipation

When It's Flowing

Your hands and feet are warm. Your skin is elastic and clear. You feel alert but not wired. Fluids move. Waste clears. You feel a natural sense of circulation through your body, your thoughts, even your emotions.

3. Regulation | The Insulation

Every system needs boundaries. In the body, that job belongs to your cell membranes. Thin but vital, they surround each cell, acting like the insulating rubber coating on an electrical wire. They choose what enters, what stays out, and how fast things move. They're selective, responsive, and dynamic like finely tuned gates. Regulation is how your body keeps order.

The Disconnect

When membranes are inflamed or degraded, they become porous. Charge leaks, toxins slip in, signals get scrambled. Chronic stress, processed food, chemicals, and gut irritation wear down the gates.

You feel puffy or reactive. Skin flares. Bloating after meals. Brain fog. You might swing between high and low energy. You feel like your system can't regulate, like everything's too much.

How It Can Show Up

When cells lose their insulation, signals can't land and the membranes leak. The following conditions show how broken regulation may appear.

- IBS and Leaky Gut
- Food Sensitivities
- Allergies
- Eczema, Dermatitis, Psoriasis
- Asthma and Allergic Rhinitis
- Autoimmune Conditions
- Migraines
- Hormone Resistance

When It's Flowing

You feel stable. Clear-minded. Have steady energy. Your skin is calm, digestion smooth, and you recover quickly after stress. Your hormones function. Immune system is kept in check. Your body responds well to input without overreacting. There's a sense of containment without overwhelm.

> ### What is Hormone Resistance?
>
> Hormone resistance happens when your body sends a message, but your cells don't hear it. It's not that your hormones are broken. It's that the gates they're trying to activate are inflamed, blocked, or too tired to respond.
>
> Think of insulin, for example. Its job is to help sugar move out of your blood and into your cells. But when your membranes are swollen or damaged, the signal can't land. So the body thinks it needs to shout louder and more insulin gets released. The same can happen with leptin (which helps you feel full and burn fat), and cortisol (which helps you handle stress).
>
> The real issue isn't always hormone production, it's hormone sensitivity and communication. And communication depends on healthy membranes. When the cell membranes calm, the gates respond. The messages start landing again. And your body can stop shouting and start listening.

A Deeper Dive | When the Cell Membranes Break Down

One of the most fragile points in your circuit is the insulation. Health problems may look different on the surface depending on which cells have leaky membranes, but the pattern beneath is the same. It isn't hundreds of separate diseases. It's the circuit breaking in different areas of the body. That's why so many conditions overlap.

Table: When the Cell Membrane Breaks Down | The table that follows shows what may happen when different cell membranes lose their insulation. It's not a diagnostic tool - it's simply a way to see how the same thread of dysfunction can appear across many systems. The goal isn't to fear the names, but to notice the pattern beneath. Always speak with your practitioner if you're managing a diagnosis.

	Weak Membrane	May Contribute To
Brain Cells	Overactivation Inflammation	Brain Fog, Alzheimer's, Parkinson's, Mood Disorders
Cardiac Cells	Electrical instability Impaired contraction	Arrhythmias, Palpitations, Fatigue
Airway Cells	Increased permeability Immune overreaction	Asthma, Chronic Sinusitis, Environmental Sensitivity
Gut Lining Cells	Barrier breakdown Immune stimulation	Leaky Gut Syndrome, Crohn's, Ulcerative Colitis,
Blood Vessel Wall Cells	Stiffening Inflammation	High Blood Pressure, Atherosclerosis, Migraines
Muscle Cells	Weak contractions Energy depletion	Fibromyalgia, Chronic Pain, CFS, Exercise Intolerance
Fat Cells	Insulin resistance Inflammation	Type 2 Diabetes, Metabolic Syndrome
Skin Cells	Moisture loss Immune reactivity	Eczema, Dermatitis, Psoriasis, Rosacea
Immune Cells	Misidentification of self Overreaction	Rheumatoid Arthritis, Autoimmune Diseases

Mast Cells	Signal hypersensitivity Histamine release	MCAS, Allergies, Chronic Hives, Histamine Symptoms
Multiple Cell Types	Widespread breakdown Systemic inflammation	Post-Viral Syndromes, CFS, Multi-System Sensitivities

What's Going on with Histamine and Allergies?

If you feel like you're reacting to everything. Foods, smells, weather changes. You're not imagining it. But it doesn't mean your body is attacking you. It means the membranes of your mast cells are porous and overwhelmed.

Mast cells are part of your immune system. They sit at the boundaries of your body, in the skin, the gut, the lungs, and act like lookouts. When they sense danger, they release histamine to alert the system. It's normal. The problem happens when the membranes of those cells become leaky.

When the insulation is weak, mast cells leak histamine at the slightest nudge. They react to things that aren't dangerous. It's not that your body is broken, it's that the gates are too open.

The symptoms shift depending on where the mast cells are leaking.
- **Skin |** Itching, rashes, hives.
- **Gut |** Bloating, nausea, loose stools.
- **Brain |** Anxiety, brain fog, insomnia,
- **Blood Vessels |** Migraines, dizziness, low blood pressure.
- **Respiratory |** Sinus congestion, hay fever, asthma.
- **Multiple Systems |** Mast cell activation syndrome (MCAS)

4. Conversion | The Engine

This is the layer where input becomes usable power. Where food and breath get turned into energy you can feel. It happens in your mitochondria - tiny engines tucked inside nearly every cell. These engines make something called ATP, the molecule your body uses to do everything. It's what lets you move, think, create, recover, and respond with strength instead of strain. Without this layer, input just sits there. But when it's working, your body lights up.

The Disconnect

Too much stress, the wrong diet, poor sleep, toxins, and chronic inflammation all wear out the engines. Instead of converting, they start to stall. You're still eating, breathing, and moving, but energy's not in abundance.

You feel tired after meals. You crash in the afternoons. Exercise feels draining instead of energising. You might feel foggy, cold, or heavy. Nothing seems particularly "off," but nothing is firing either.

How It Can Show Up

When the engines stall, fuel isn't turned into power. The following conditions show how broken conversion may appear in the body.

- o Chronic Fatigue Syndrome
- o Brain Fog and Slow Thinking
- o Premature Ageing
- o Depression
- o Heart Failure
- o Neurodegeneration

When It's Flowing

You feel charged, not overstimulated, just steady. You move easily, recover quickly, and think clearly. Your metabolism feels responsive. Your body feels warm from within. There's power behind your actions.

A Deeper Dive | When the Mitochondria Power Down

At the centre of almost every modern health struggle is one common theme - the body's engines, the mitochondria, begin to fail. The conditions vary. Fatigue, gut issues, heart problems, muscle weakness. Because different cells have different functions. But beneath it all, the pattern is the same - poor energy conversion.

Table: When the Mitochondria Power Down | The following table shows how mitochondrial slowdown can ripple through the body. You'll notice a lot of similarities with the cell membrane table. That's because mitochondria and membranes are not separate problems. They're two sides of the same coin. One failure feeds the other. Remember, these aren't direct causes, just patterns seen. Always speak with your practitioner if you're managing a diagnosis.

	When Mitochondria Slow	May Contribute To
Brain Cells	Low energy output Neuroinflammation	Depression, Anxiety, Brain Fog, Alzheimer's, Parkinson's
Cardiac Cells	Energy deficit Weak contractility	Arrhythmias, Heart Failure, Cardiomyopathy

Gut Cells	Low enzyme output Barrier dysfunction	Crohn's, Ulcerative Colitis, Leaky Gut Syndrome
Blood Vessel Wall Cells	Poor vascular tone Poor vascular perfusion	Raynaud's, Hypertension, Circulatory Issues, POTS
Muscle Cells	Reduced endurance Slow recovery	Fibromyalgia, CFS, Exercise Intolerance
Skin Cells	Slow healing Collagen loss	Delayed Wound Healing, Acne, Premature Ageing
Reproductive Cells	Hormone disruption	PCOS, Menstrual Disorders, Low Testosterone, Infertility
Endometrial Cells	Inflammation Poor cell turnover	Endometriosis, Pelvic Pain Syndromes
Bone Cells	Weak turnover Reduced mineralisation	Osteopenia, Osteoporosis, Delayed Fracture Healing
Immune Cells	Poor response Dysregulated	Recurring Infections Autoimmune Conditions
Cancer Cells	Cells bypass natural death Altered energy pathways	Mitochondrial dysfunction is frequently found in cancer

5. Expression | The Output Channels

Expression is how energy (ATP) is used. Some flows outward - into movement, speech, and thought. Some flows inward - into hormones, repair, and healing. Either way, energy isn't meant to sit still. It wants to move, to be expressed. These are your output channels. When expression is clear, nothing stagnates. Energy turns into action, and repair can take its course.

The Disconnect

Sometimes there's too much coming in - noise, light, demands, stimulation - and the system gets flooded. Other times, the outlets shrink. You don't move, you don't speak, you hold back what you feel.

When expression is jammed or overwhelmed, energy doesn't get used the way it should. Outwardly, it can leave you restless, tense, or stuck. You speak too much, or not at all. Inwardly, it means repair slows. Hormones slip out of balance. Inflammation lingers. And healing never quite finishes. Fuel is there, but it isn't being used.

How It Can Show Up

When the output channels jam or overload, signals build without release. The following conditions show how blocked expression can show up.

- Anxiety and Panic Attacks
- Muscle Tension
- Hormone Imbalance
- Speech Blocks
- Tension Headaches
- Jaw Clenching (Bruxism)
- Sensory Overload
- Slow Healing and Repair

When It's Flowing

Your body moves freely. Your speech is clear, steady, and honest. Emotions flow without overwhelming. Inwardly, repair and balance hum in the background. You feel a natural rhythm between input and output, nothing feels forced, nothing feels stuck.

6. Protection | The Shield

Protection isn't about being tough. It's about keeping what's yours in, and what's not, out. Your body has built-in layers to help with that.

- **Fascia |** Holds your form and keeps everything in its place.
  (If this is new, see "More Than Connective Tissue" on page 23)
- **Biofield |** Helps shield and protect your circuit.
  (If this is new, see "Where There's Charge, There's a Field" on page 25)

When these layers are working well, you feel clear. You know what's yours to carry and what isn't. You can move through the world without getting overwhelmed. But when they're worn down, it's harder to tell. Everything starts to blur. You might feel scattered, heavy, or drained, and not know why. This layer of your circuit is about boundaries. It helps you stay steady, stay centred, and stay you.

The Disconnect

Tight fascia, chronic tension, and trauma - compress the circuit. You lose flexibility. Signals get scrambled. The system gets hypersensitive or numb. Your shield starts to fail, and you feel it all.

You flinch easily. You feel wired, shaky, or like you're too reactive. Your body feels stiff, like you're bracing all the time. Even rest doesn't feel safe.

How It Can Show Up

When the body's shield fails, tissues lose support. The following conditions show how broken protection can appear in the body. These patterns aren't for diagnosis, just a way of seeing how the body may respond.

- Chronic Muscle Pain
- Chronic Stiffness
- Fibromyalgia
- Environmental Sensitivities
- Energy Drain in Crowds
- Chronic Fatigue

Fascia | More Than Connective Tissue

Fascia is the connective tissue that wraps around everything inside your body - your muscles, bones, nerves, and organs. It holds everything together. But it's not just packaging. Fascia is alive.

It senses. It responds. It distributes force, hydration, and even electrical signals. It's made mostly of water, which holds shape, tension, and even traces of past stress. Yes, fascia holds memory. That's why old emotions can resurface during movement or massage.

When it's tight, dry, or tangled, everything feels stiff, sore, or blocked. Pain often starts in the fascia long before it shows up in a scan. Care for your fascia, and your whole body flows and moves with ease.

When It's Flowing

You feel safe in your own skin. Pressure doesn't instantly penetrate. You recover quickly after stress. Your body feels light but contained. Boundaries are clear, what's yours stays yours, and you don't absorb everything around you.

Reading the Body Through Fascia

These patterns aren't prescriptive, but they can help you see your body as more than structure. As a living map of what's been carried. And what may be ready to move.

	What You Might Notice	Patterns Often Observed
Cranial Fascia	Headaches, Dizziness, Jaw Pain	Overthinking, sensory overload, held expression
Neck & Throat Fascia	Hoarseness, Anxiety, Neck Pain	Words unspoken, swallowed emotion, fear of being seen
Chest Fascia	Breathlessness, Panic, Poor Posture	Grief, heartbreak, protection, longing
Diaphragm Fascia	Anxiety, Shallow Breath, Reflux	Unprocessed fear, held alertness, freeze response
Abdominal Fascia	Constipation, Bloating	Control, hidden shame
Pelvic Fascia	Period Pain, Painful Sex, Pelvic Tension	Safety, power, hidden trauma, boundary breaches
Spinal Fascia	Sciatica, Back Pain, Muscle Tightness	Responsibility, bracing, identity load

Biofield | Where There's Charge, There's a Field

Your body isn't just chemical - it's electrical. And wherever there's electrical flow, there's a magnetic field. It's not theory, and it's not a new idea - it's physics. Every wire that carries current produces a field around it - so does your body.

This field, often called the biofield, influences how you sense, protect, and respond. Its strength depends on your electrical flow. The steadier your circuit, the more charge moves, and the stronger the biofield becomes.

It's not abstract. It's measurable. Your heart and brain produce the strongest electromagnetic fields in your body. Medicine relies on this every day - an ECG traces the heart's electrical activity, an EEG records brainwaves. Advanced tools like MEG and MCG even measure the magnetic fields those currents create, without touching the body.

You've probably felt the biofield without realising - the sense of someone walking into a room before you see them. Or feeling "off" in yourself when another person is unsettled.

This book won't dwell on the biofield, and you don't need to know all the details. The point is simple. Your body isn't just chemical - it's electric. And the field around you is proof of that.

7. Reset | The Return Path

Reset is your body's return path. It's how the system rests and releases. Every circuit needs a way to close the loop, to discharge what's done and make space for the next cycle. In your body, reset means sleep, elimination, and stillness. It tells your cells it's safe to stop, to rest, to breathe. Releasing what isn't needed and anchoring what is. Without it, everything builds up.

The Disconnect

No sleep rhythm. No rest rhythm. And no eating rhythm. Life stretches too long. The day blurs into night. The pause disappears. And your body forgets how to end a cycle. So, it just keeps going until it crashes.

You're always on. Even in the dark, your brain won't stop. You feel wired. Restless. Broken sleep. Tension stuck in the tissues. Your body clenches, because it never gets to let go.

How It Can Show Up

When the return path fails, reset and repair is lost. The following conditions show how a broken return path may appear in the body.

- Trouble Falling Asleep
- Waking Unrefreshed
- Inability to Fully Relax
- Feeling "Wired but Tired"
- Burnout or Adrenal Fatigue
- Tension Headaches
- Sensory Overload
- Anxiety and Restlessness

When It's Flowing

You sleep deeply. You wake clear. Digestion flows. Your mind pauses between thoughts. You can stop working without guilt. You rest without needing distraction. There's a grounded stillness inside you that doesn't reach for stimulation.

Questionnaire | Mapping Where You Are

On the following pages, you'll see two short checklists for every layer. One showing common signs of strain when the flow is disrupted. And one showing signs of repair when the current is strong.

This isn't about labels or diagnosis. It's about recognising patterns. Notice where you tick the most, and where you barely mark anything. Both matter.

If you'd like, date your notes. As you work through the Six-Phase Reset, you may be surprised how many boxes shift from strain to repair.

Signs of Strain

Tick anything that feels familiar, even if it's just now and then.

1. Reception | The Solar Panels

- ☐ I wake up groggy, even after 7 - 8 hours of sleep.
- ☐ I rely on coffee or stimulants to "switch on" in the morning.
- ☐ I spend most of the day indoors under artificial light.
- ☐ My mood dips in Winter or on cloudy days.
- ☐ My skin feels dull, flat, or lifeless.

2. Transmission | The Wires

- ☐ I often feel thirsty, even when drinking plenty.
- ☐ I get dizzy when standing quickly.
- ☐ My skin, eyes, or mouth often feel dry.
- ☐ I have issues with constipation or headaches.
- ☐ I get cramps, restless legs, or have circulation problems.

3. Regulation | The Insulation

- ☐ My energy swings high and low during the day.
- ☐ I often bloat, flush, or react after meals.
- ☐ I have ongoing skin issues (eczema, hives, dermatitis).
- ☐ I notice seasonal allergies, hay fever, or asthma flare-ups.
- ☐ I've been told I have food sensitivities or an autoimmune condition.

4. Conversion | The Engine

- ☐ Exercise leaves me drained instead of refreshed.

- ☐ I struggle with cold hands and feet or feeling "cold inside."
- ☐ I've experienced brain fog, memory slips, or low focus.
- ☐ I've noticed slow healing, premature ageing, or recurring fatigue.
- ☐ My health feels confusing, like lots of different issues without a clear cause.

5. Expression | The Output Channels

- ☐ I often feel anxious, tense, or restless.
- ☐ I clench my jaw, grind my teeth, or hold tension in my body.
- ☐ My speech feels blocked, I hold back what I want to say.
- ☐ My body holds tension when I don't move or express myself.
- ☐ I feel overloaded by noise, light, or sensory input.

6. Protection | The Shield

- ☐ I feel drained or heavy after being around groups of people.
- ☐ My muscles and fascia feel tight, stiff, or painful.
- ☐ I'm highly sensitive to environments, like I take on too much.
- ☐ Even at rest, I feel on edge or braced, like I can't fully relax.
- ☐ Stress or trauma seems to stay stuck in my body.

7. Reset | The Return Path

- ☐ I have trouble falling asleep or wake a lot during the night.
- ☐ I feel wired and unable to fully relax.
- ☐ I struggle to stop working without guilt or distraction.
- ☐ I reach for stimulation (scrolling, snacking, noise) instead of resting.
- ☐ I often wake with tension headaches or a restless mind.

Signs of Repair

Return to these as you move through the Six-Phase Reset.

1. Reception | The Solar Panels

- ☐ I wake with energy and don't need stimulants to start my day.
- ☐ Light lifts my mood and focus almost instantly.
- ☐ My skin looks bright and feels alive.
- ☐ I feel connected to time, seasons, and the world around me.
- ☐ I sense an inner spark, like my body is charged.

2. Transmission | The Wires

- ☐ My hands and feet are warm, even in cooler weather.
- ☐ My skin feels elastic and hydrated. My eyes look clear and bright.
- ☐ I rarely get dizzy or foggy.
- ☐ Digestion and elimination feel smooth and regular.
- ☐ I feel well-hydrated without constantly needing to sip water.

3. Regulation | The Insulation

- ☐ My digestion feels calm and steady.
- ☐ My skin is clear and rarely inflamed.
- ☐ My immune system feels balanced, and not overreactive.
- ☐ I have steady, predictable energy through the day.
- ☐ My body responds to food, environment, and stress, without extremes.

4. Conversion | The Engine

- ☐ I have consistent energy and don't suffer from afternoon dips.

- ☐ Movement and exercise give me more energy than they take.
- ☐ My body feels warm from within even on cold days.
- ☐ I recover quickly from injury and illness.
- ☐ My thoughts are clear, focused, and steady.

5. Expression | The Output Channels

- ☐ My body moves easily and doesn't hold tension.
- ☐ My speech feels honest, clear, and unforced.
- ☐ My emotions flow without overwhelming me.
- ☐ My hormones feel balanced and recovery feels natural.
- ☐ My output matches my input. Nothing feels blocked or excessive.

6. Protection | The Shield

- ☐ I feel safe in my body.
- ☐ Stress moves through me without lingering.
- ☐ My muscles and fascia feel supple.
- ☐ I can be around people without feeling drained.
- ☐ I know what's mine to carry, and I can let go of the rest.

7. Reset | The Return Path

- ☐ I fall asleep easily and wake feeling clear.
- ☐ I can pause without guilt and enjoy stillness.
- ☐ Detox, and elimination flow naturally.
- ☐ My mind finds quiet space between thoughts.
- ☐ I feel rested, grounded, and ready for what's next.

The Body as a Circuit | Summary

When the circuit hums, you feel steady. When it kinks, jams, or frays, that's when dysfunction begins. What looks like a thousand different diseases is often just one truth - the current has broken somewhere. The way back isn't to fight the label, but to find the kink in the circuit and restore it.

And that's what comes next. The Seven Pillars of Health are how you repair the circuit. They're the fuels and rhythms your body has always run on. When they return, the current returns. And the body remembers how to heal.

The Seven
Pillars of Health

The Seven Pillars of Health

Health isn't built on hacks, willpower, or adding more to your to-do list - it's built on charge. These seven pillars affect how you receive, carry, and use that charge. They're the fuels your biology already knows, waiting to be uncovered.

The names may feel unusual at first: breath, light, water, land, fire, fat, rhythm. They sound almost too simple. But that's the point. Somewhere along the way, health was buried under jargon and made to sound complex. These words bring it back to what's real and obvious. Simple fuels. Simple rhythms.

Each one supports several layers of the circuit at once. Each one brings back a piece of the map you were never meant to lose.

1. Breath

Breath regulates the whole system. It moves charge, calms the body, and controls rhythm. It's the first signal of life and the forgotten foundation of health.

2. Light

Light fuels your cells and tells your body what time it is. It sets your biological clock, powers the mitochondria and regulates hormones.

3. Water

Water shapes your structure, carries charge, and allows energy to flow smoothly through the system. Without water, the circuit runs dry.

4. Land

Where you live, what you touch, and what surrounds you - all of it shapes your circuit. A healthy environment nourishes the flow, while a stressed one can interrupt it.

5. Fire

Fire represents the spark in your mitochondria - the body's engines. When they burn clean, energy flows, recovery comes naturally, and your body feels steady.

6. Fat

Saturated fats (the ones solid at room temperature) hold efficient slow-burning energy. They stabilise your system, form your cell membranes, fuel the fire, and give you resilience and stamina.

7. Rhythm

Rhythm holds the whole thing together. It's not just what you do, but when you do it. Timing restores function and keeps the system from overloading.

1. Breath

Before hunger, before light, your body knew breath. Not as effort. Not as skill. But as rhythm.

You weren't taught to breathe. You remembered. Breath came before the world made noise. It came before the mind made demands. And it's still here. Beneath the tension. Beneath the holding. Quiet. Waiting.

The Function

Breath holds your whole system, it sparks the fire, and it guides the return. When breath is steady, full, and unforced, it signals safety to every layer of the body. Muscles release. Nerves settle. Digestion restarts. Your posture finds centre. Your system shifts from defence to calm.

Breath Primarily Fuels Three Layers of the Body's Circuit

Conversion | The Engine - Breath draws oxygen into the lungs and feeds the mitochondria. This is where energy is made. Without breath, there is no power.

Expression | The Output Channels - Every movement, every word, every release rides on breath. Breath lets the body speak.

Reset | The Return Path - A slow, complete exhale helps the body downshift. It guides charge out. It makes space. It resets the nervous system and says, "You're safe now."

The Fracture

We lost our breath when we rushed. When we braced, clenched, scrolled, and hurried through noise and deadlines. Tension set in, and the breath rose high in the chest instead of grounded in the belly.

We sigh. Gasp. Yawn. Trying to catch up without realising we never fully exhaled. It's not your fault. But it matters. Tension in your breath becomes tension in your life. You're not broken. You're just disconnected from your first rhythm.

Restored in Phases 1, 3 & 4

2. Light

You don't see light. You receive it. It enters your body as signal. It tells your cells what time it is, what task to do, and what rhythm to follow. Light doesn't just brighten the world outside you, it aligns the world inside you.

Your eyes are not just for vision. They are clocks. Your skin is not just a covering. It's a solar panel. Your body listens for light. And when the signal is steady, you steady too.

The Function

Light governs the rhythm of your entire body. When light enters your system at the right time and in the right form it switches everything on. It whispers, "Now," and your body remembers what to do.

- Morning light stirs the system ... "Wake."
- Midday light powers it ... "Go."
- Evening light winds it down ... "Release."
- Darkness rebuilds what the day used ... "Return."

Light Primarily Fuels Five Layers of the Body's Circuit

Reception | The Solar Panels - Light enters through the eyes and skin. It charges the circuit and sets your body's clock.

Conversion | The Engine - Light at the molecular level spins the mitochondrial engine. Without light, the engine can't efficiently convert fuel into ATP.

Expression | The Output Channels - Light guides how your cells and body use energy, shaping mood, hormones, and daily rhythm.

Protection | The Shield - Energy from light strengthens your biofield and charges your fascia. Light helps form the shield around the circuit.

Reset | The Return Path - As light fades, your body prepares to return. It slows, recalibrates, and begins its rebuild. Ready to receive again.

The Fracture

Modern life has blocked the signal. We wake in the dark, skip the sunrise, sit under artificial lights, and scroll through the day. Our body, confused, lost its pulse. Sleep becomes shallow. Hormones drift. Appetite and mood slide off track. Energy feels flat as the mitochondria slow. We weren't made to live cut off from nature. But the light was dimmed, and the body forgot what time it is.

Restored in Phases 1, 2 & 4

3. Water

Water is more than a drink - it's the medium your whole body depends on. It fills your blood, cells, and fascia, cushions your joints, and lines your mitochondria. But for it to do its job well, the kind of water matters.

Your body needs water that can hold and carry charge. That means water that is *structured*, *mineralised*, and *flowing*. Structured water forms when it's exposed to light, minerals, and motion. This kind of water stabilises tissues and keeps energy smooth.

If you take in plenty of water but still feel stiff, tired, or foggy, the issue may not be how much you drink, but about quality and movement.

The Function

Water doesn't just fill space - it shapes how your body works. In fascia, it lets layers glide instead of sticking. Around joints, it cushions impact and prevents grinding. In the mitochondria, it forms a lining that supports the conversion of fuel into ATP.

When your water is structured and mineral-rich, these systems stay supple and responsive. Movement feels smooth, recovery comes easier, and energy production runs without friction.

Water Primarily Fuels Three Layers of the Body's Circuit

Transmission | The Wires - Water is the highway for charge. It moves through your blood, fascia, and tissues. Ensuring nutrients and energy reach where they belong.

Conversion | The Engine - Water helps the mitochondria move energy. Without it, fat can't burn, oxygen can't be used, and the fire can't ignite.

Protection | The Shield - Water hydrates the fascia. Healthy fascia supports the body and carries signal.

The Fracture

We dried out slowly. Not just our skin, but our charge. Air got dry. Water and salt were skipped. Movement disappeared. And the water inside us slowed.

Our fascia tightened. Our thinking dulled. Dehydration doesn't always show as thirst. It can feel like headaches, or tightness, or fatigue that doesn't make sense. Or sometimes, you just feel "off."

Restored in Phases 1 & 5

4. Land

The land isn't just background. It shapes you. Guides you. Charges or drains you. Where you live, what you breathe, what surrounds you, even the microbes in your gut - it all speaks. The nervous system listens constantly. Your body hears it before you do.

This pillar is not about becoming afraid of your environment. It's about remembering that you're part of it. That it shapes you, guides how safe you feel, and that your system can return to peace when your space becomes still again.

The Function

Your environment is the quiet voice your biology never stops listening to. It tells you when to brace. And it tells you when to release. Before you speak, before you move, your body already knows the room. If it's calm and clean, your system opens. If it's noisy, jagged, or synthetic, your system tightens.

- A quiet space says ... "You can rest now."
- Natural light says ... "This place is alive."
- Clutter and chemicals say ... "Stay alert."
- Living materials say ... "You belong."

Land Primarily Fuels Three Layers of the Body's Circuit

Regulation | The Insulation - The environment affects how well your cell membranes hold charge. Toxins cause swelling and leaking in the membranes. Clean, calm spaces help cells seal again so your circuit can stabilise.

Protection | The Shield - Natural materials, clean air, light, and calm support your fascia and biofield. They send a message, "You're safe." That one signal alone can help healing begin.

Reset | The Return Path - When your space is still, your body stops bracing, and you come out of defence. The system exhales and detox pathways open. You can finally rest and reset.

The Fracture

We stopped building with intention. The materials changed. The air changed. The light changed. But your body didn't. Now we live in boxes full of signals our nervous system doesn't know how to understand. Artificial light and flickering screens. Clutter and overstimulation. Mould, dust, and stale air. No connection to the outdoors. It all adds up. Even when you try to rest, your body keeps hearing, "Stay alert."

Restored in Phase 3

5. Fire

You don't notice when it first begins. Just a yawn too early in the day. The quiet fade of motivation. A sense that something's "off," even when all the tests say you're fine. This pillar is for the ones who kept going. Who called it stress. Or age. Or weakness. But really, your fire dimmed.

Food and oxygen alone don't guarantee energy. They're the raw materials. But to actually burn them into usable power, your mitochondria need the right spark and conditions. That's the fire.

Mitochondria are tuned by light, by temperature, by the timing of your day, by the quality of your water, and even by how much you rest between bursts of activity. When those signals are right, the burn is clean. Energy flows easily, recovery is fast, and your system feels steady.

When they're off, the fire is weak. You'll still make ATP, but it's less efficient. You get more waste, more fatigue, more inflammation. It feels like you're always running uphill.

The Function

When your mitochondria burn clean, your energy feels anchored. You think clearer. You move steadier. Repair feels natural. Healing happens quietly in the background instead of being a constant battle.

You were designed to make energy with ease. To wake up with clarity. To move through the day without dragging your body behind you. When your internal fire is strong, there's a lightness, a steadiness, a glow about you.

Fire Primarily Fuels Two Layers of the Body's Circuit

Conversion | The Engine - Mitochondria take the raw fuels of food and oxygen and, with a strong fire, burn them to make ATP.

Expression | The Output Channels - Once energy is made, the body uses it. Thought, speech, digestion, healing. They all depend on mitochondrial function.

Losing Power

Mitochondrial decline creeps in, so slowly, that most people don't notice until they're deep in it. These stages are not strict numbers, but they show the kind of drift many people experience on the way towards burnout.

10% Loss | You just feel a little "off." Afternoon dips. Focus drifts. You can still push through with coffee or carbs, but it costs more effort than it used to.

30% Loss | Energy dips turn into crashes. Sleep feels light, unrefreshing. Gut issues surface. Memory slips. You start to feel like you're ageing faster than you should.

50% Loss | You wake already tired. Mood fluctuates more easily. Cravings rise. Hormones feel unstable. You feel less steady in yourself, less at home in your body.

70% Loss | Fatigue is constant now. Inflammation hums in the background. Illnesses feel confusing, and unexplained. Pain rises. Life feels harder than it should.

... Continued

90% Loss | The system grows dim. Speech slows. Fatigue becomes crushing. Bed is a necessity, not choice. It feels like your body is shutting down.

You're not stuck here. With the right inputs, the body can rebuild.

The Fracture

In the world you live in now, your mitochondria are under constant attack, not from a single enemy, but from a thousand small ones. Artificial light and screens late into the evening. Processed foods and oils that inflame. Days spent sitting indoors without movement or sun. Shallow sleep that never reaches repair. Stress that never lets go. Your mitochondria were built to adapt, but not without limit. Over time the fire dims, the engine slows.

Restored in Phases 1, 2, 4 & 5

6. Fat

You weren't made to run on fumes. You were made to burn clean. To be steady, strong, and sustained by something deeper than snacks, coffee, or carbs.

This pillar is for those tired of the crash. The spike, then the fall. The grazing all day, but still feeling empty. The bodies stuck in sugar loops, jittery, wired, but never satisfied.

The Function

Saturated fat is your slow-burning fuel. When your body runs on clean fat, things calm. Blood sugar stays balanced. Cravings ease. Hormones begin to settle. Your brain feels clearer and less reactive. You stop chasing energy hits and start moving with ease. There's calm in your system again.

Fat Primarily Fuels Three Layers of the Body's Circuit

Regulation | The Insulation - Saturated fat stabilises your cell membranes by stopping leaks, and keeping order inside and out.

Conversion | The Engine - Mitochondria turn fat into energy. Unlike quick sugars, saturated fat burns slowly and cleanly. Providing smooth and stable energy without the crashes.

Expression | The Output Channels - Fat is the backbone for many hormones and for rebuilding tissues. With the right fats, your body can signal clearly, repair smoothly, and keep expression steady.

The Fracture

Most people are stuck in sugar mode. Constant snacking, processed foods, hidden sugars in meals and drinks. Low-fat diets that strip the body of what it needs. It all adds up. Over time the body forgets how to burn fat. And the mitochondrial fire dims.

Restored in Phase 5

Why the Type of Fat Matters

Not all fats are the same. Some strengthen your system. Others make it fragile and leaky. Choose fats that are stable and hold.

Saturated Fats | Stable Fat - Tallow, butter, ghee. Animal fats. Fats solid at room temperature. They resist damage. They burn clean. They strengthen your cell membranes and help stabilise the circuit.

Polyunsaturated Fats | Fragile Fat - Seed oils, canola oil, soybean oil, sunflower oil, vegetable oil, even margarine. They all break down easily, especially when heated. When these unstable fats are built into your cell membranes, your cells become fragile, dysregulated, and start to leak.

For a refresher on cell membranes and what happens when they become leaky, see "Regulation / The Insulation" on pages 13 - 16.

7. Rhythm

There's something your body is always listening for, even if you're not aware of it. A quiet pattern underneath everything. Some people call it routine. Others call it structure. But rhythm is more than that.

It's the timing your body was built to follow. The pauses between. The space to breathe. When that rhythm is in place, life flows. You sleep when it's time to sleep. You feel hungry when it's time to eat. You move when it's time to move. And you rest, deeply, when it's time to rest.

The Function

1. Daily Rhythm | Your Circadian Clock

This is your 24-hour light-dark cycle. It tells your cells what to do and when to do it. Morning light starts the day's programs. Darkness prepares you for rest and repair. Disrupt this rhythm, and your energy, sleep, hormones, digestion, and mood all suffer. Restore it, and everything begins to fall back into place.

2. Weekly Rhythm | Your Recovery Pattern

You were never meant to operate at full speed seven days a week. You need a rhythm of exertion and rest. A reliable point where your body and nervous system know it's safe to relax, reset, and recover. It means scheduling space. Time without screens, silence between commitments, nature instead of stimulation. A reset day once a week isn't indulgent, it's essential.

3. Seasonal Rhythm | Your Seasonal Alignment

Each season brings different light, temperature, foods, emotions, and movement. Your biology changes with it whether you realise it or not. In Summer, your body wants light, movement, energy. In Winter, it craves warmth, stillness, and deeper rest. But most people treat every month the same and wonder why they feel off.

What Each Season Signals

Your body doesn't guess the season. It knows, by light. Each day, the amount, angle, and wavelength (colour) of light hitting your eyes sends a message straight to your brain's internal clock. As the light shifts with each season, your body is designed to shift too.

1. Spring | The Reawakening

Spring brings more light, and with it, a quiet stirring from within. As the days lengthen, mood lifts, energy returns, and the body begins to awaken from Winter. Mitochondria start ramping up again, preparing for movement. Hormones like cortisol and thyroid gently rise. This is the season of new energy, of clearing the fog, of remembering what it feels like to begin again.

2. Summer | The Peak

Summer is the height of the year, full light, full power. Sunlight pours in, raising serotonin, vitamin D, and the desire to act, move, and create. If you rise with the sun and move in the mornings, your mitochondria burn hot, fuelling strength, focus, and expression. Libido, mental energy, and clarity often peak here. This is the season to build, to do, to speak. Not from force, but from fullness. Summer is when the body wants to shine.

3. Autumn | The Pull Inward

Autumn draws you inward. The light softens, melatonin arrives earlier, and energy begins to settle. You might notice your appetite shift slightly, your body preparing for the colder months ahead. The thyroid quiets, the nervous system slows, and the desire to do gives way to the need to reflect. It's not collapse, it's compression. A gentle grounding. This is the season of holding what matters, letting go of what doesn't, and allowing stillness to return in small ways.

4. Winter | The Resting

Winter is not a failure of energy, it's the wisdom of rest. The days shorten. Light retreats. And your body follows. Metabolism slows. Mitochondria shift from growth to repair. Fat loss pauses, not because you're broken, but because this is how life restores itself. You may crave more sleep, simplicity, warmth, or quiet. Winter is the season of deep alignment, where the body returns to its roots and prepares, patiently, for what's next.

Rhythm Primarily Fuels Four Layers of the Body's Circuit

Reception | The Solar Panels - Rhythm begins with receiving. Your body notices these cues and recognises time. This sets the tone for everything that follows.

Conversion | The Engine - When energy is made and when it's used is guided by rhythm. It tells your mitochondria when to fire and when to rest.

Expression | The Output Channels - Hormone release, repair, even thought and movement all follow these clocks. They tell the body not just what to do, but when to do it.

Reset | The Return Path - Rhythm creates space for the exhale. It guides your body into balance. It tells you when it's safe to stop and how to come back to stillness.

The Fracture

Modern life runs on artificial time. We wake with alarms, work under constant light, eat at odd hours, and stay up too late. Climate control confuses the season. Summer foods are eaten year-round. Days are packed without pause, weeks without rest, seasons without shift. And the body, pushed out of its design, loses its beat.

Restored in Phases 2 & 6

Questionnaire | Mapping Where You Are

The coming pages will help you notice where your health is strong, and where it's asking for help. You'll see two checklists - one for signs of strain and disruption, and one for signs of repair and rhythm. This is not about judgement. It's about noticing what's calling for attention.

Consider dating any marks you make, so that as you move through the Six-Phase Reset, you can look back and see how far you've come.

Signs of Strain

Tick anything that feels familiar, even if it's just now and then.

1. Breath

- ☐ I hold my breath without realising, especially under stress.
- ☐ I breathe mostly through my mouth, not my nose.
- ☐ I often sigh, yawn, or feel short of breath during the day.
- ☐ I breathe in my upper chest, not belly - my breath feels shallow.
- ☐ I lose touch with my breath in moments I need it most.

2. Light

- ☐ I miss the sunrise or don't see the morning sky.
- ☐ I spend most of my day indoors or under artificial light.
- ☐ I feel groggy or heavy during the day.
- ☐ I use screens late at night or fall asleep near devices.
- ☐ My sleep is delayed, broken, or I feel wired at night.

3. Water

- ☐ I don't drink enough clean water, or I forget until I'm already thirsty.
- ☐ I've been on a low-salt diet and feel flat or depleted.
- ☐ My skin or lips feel dry and my eyes sting or blur.
- ☐ I crave salty foods or feel faint when standing.
- ☐ Water seems to pass straight through me instead of replenishing me.

4. Land

- ☐ I feel overstimulated in noisy or artificial spaces.

- ☐ I rarely touch earth, sand, stone, or grass with bare feet.
- ☐ I feel foggy or drained when indoors for too long.
- ☐ My home doesn't feel grounded, calming, or restful.
- ☐ I avoid going outside unless I have to.

5. Fire

- ☐ I feel unmotivated or tired, no matter how much I rest.
- ☐ I start things strong, but can't sustain them.
- ☐ My body temperature feels unstable (cold hands and feet).
- ☐ I crave stimulants (coffee, sugar) just to feel alive.
- ☐ I rely on intensity (exercise, stress, adrenaline) to spark momentum.

6. Fat

- ☐ I feel hungry often, or unsatisfied after eating, so often snack.
- ☐ My energy crashes mid-morning or mid-afternoon.
- ☐ My skin, nails, or hair feel dry, brittle, or dull.
- ☐ I crave sugar or carbs to get through the day.
- ☐ I forget or avoid including saturated fats in my meals.

7. Rhythm

- ☐ My sleep and mealtimes shift randomly through the week.
- ☐ I feel out of sync with the day or season.
- ☐ I skip rest, or overwork without noticing, until I crash.
- ☐ I rush from one thing to the next and forget to breathe.
- ☐ I've lost touch with when to stop, or how to recover.

Signs of Repair

Return to these as you move through the Six-Phase Reset.

1. Breath

- ☐ You breathe mostly through your nose, even while walking.
- ☐ Your chest feels open, and your ribs can expand with ease.
- ☐ You return to your breath in moments of stress.
- ☐ You feel grounded and calm before reacting.
- ☐ You notice your breath often throughout the day.

2. Light

- ☐ You get morning light, and you feel the sun anchor your days.
- ☐ You naturally feel sleepy when the light dims in the evenings.
- ☐ You fall asleep easily and wake with steady energy.
- ☐ You crave time outside and feel better after it.
- ☐ You instinctively turn off screens or dim lights at night.

3. Water

- ☐ You feel hydrated without needing constant sips.
- ☐ Your lips, skin, and eyes feel naturally moist.
- ☐ You don't get dizzy when you stand quickly.
- ☐ You feel refreshed and clear-headed after drinking.
- ☐ Water seems to nourish you, not just flush through.

4. Land

- ☐ You feel clearer and calmer after stepping outside.

- [ ] You notice the weather and subtle outdoor shifts.
- [ ] Your home or workspace feels peaceful and ordered.
- [ ] You feel grounded.
- [ ] You naturally seek nature, even in small ways.

5. Fire

- [ ] You wake with inner energy instead of needing caffeine.
- [ ] You feel warmth in your body, not too cold, not too hot.
- [ ] You have drive without strain, motivation without stress.
- [ ] You no longer chase adrenaline to feel alive.
- [ ] You carry a stable glow, even on quiet days.

6. Fat

- [ ] You feel full and steady between meals.
- [ ] You stop chasing snacks, and your body asks for real food.
- [ ] Your hormones feel steady and regulated.
- [ ] Your energy feels calm, not scattered or depleted.
- [ ] Your skin and hair feel healthy and alive.

7. Rhythm

- [ ] You feel the rhythm of the day, when to rise, when to rest.
- [ ] You eat, move, and sleep at similar times without forcing it.
- [ ] You make space for rest and recovery without guilt.
- [ ] You feel the seasons shifting and adjust naturally.
- [ ] You don't chase time, you flow with it.

The Six-Phase
Reset

How to Walk This Path

This isn't a program. It's not a challenge. It's not a fix-everything-in-30-days system. This is a gentle return.

What you're holding isn't a rulebook. It's a rhythm, a way of living that helps you reconnect to the design already written into your body. You don't have to earn it. And you don't have to do everything at once.

Each phase will offer you anchors in the seven pillars of health: breath, light, water, land, fire, fat, and rhythm. You'll learn how to begin strengthening them in everyday life.

But this isn't about doing them all. This is about building a rhythm that lasts. Some parts you might breeze through. Some you'll sit with for weeks. That's right. That's rhythm.

Let this feel like a gentle unfolding, not another list of things you've failed to finish. If you get tired, pause. If you feel excited, run with it. If you get lost, return to breath.

Your Six-Phase Reset Journey

The journey unfolds in six phases. One at a time. Each phase prepares the body for the next. Each one clears a layer, rebuilds a part, and brings you closer to health that feels steady, strong, and yours.

There's no rush. Take the time your body needs. Don't move to the next until you complete the last. Feel the changes. Let each phase do its work. Slower is better. This is not a race.

Phase 1 | Build the Foundation

Length: ~ 4 weeks

Pillars Restored: Breath, Light, Water, Fire

This phase lays the groundwork. Before anything can be rebuilt, the body needs safety, rhythm, and charge. You'll learn how to breathe properly, receive real light, hydrate in a way your cells can use, and move in a way that restores flow. These are the first signals the body recognises. Simple, steady, and powerful.

Phase 2 | Reset the Body Clock

Length: ~ 4 weeks

Pillars Restored: Light, Fire, Rhythm

Once the body feels safe, you begin to realign with time. This phase reconnects you to natural light and darkness. The two strongest cues for healing. You'll learn how to wake with the sun, eat in time, return to darkness at night, and let your circadian rhythm take the lead. This is when sleep deepens, digestion improves, and you begin to feel truly rested again.

Phase 3 | The Right Environment

Length: ~ 4 weeks

Pillars Restored: Breath, Land

Healing needs the right environment. This phase clears what's in the way - dust, clutter, toxins, and anything else the body is quietly reacting to. You'll learn how to create a space that feels safe and clean to your nervous system.

Phase 4 | Build Your Mitochondria

Length: ~ 4 - 6 weeks

Pillars Restored: Breath, Light, Fire

Now you build strength, at the cellular level. This is where you introduce the signals that remind your mitochondria how to work: cold, restorative light and strength. It's not about pushing, it's about activating the engines inside you. You'll feel more stable, more alive, and less fragile.

Phase 5 | Fuel the Fire

Length: ~ 6 - 8 weeks

Pillars Restored: Fire, Fat

Energy depends on the right fuel. This phase shifts you away from unstable energy, processed food, and blood sugar crashes. Towards nourishment that truly sustains you. You'll learn how to eat for health, not just calories. Meals will become simpler, richer, and more satisfying. You'll feel full again. Sharp again. Fed in a way you forgot was possible.

Phase 6 | Live in Rhythm

Length: Ongoing, for life

Pillar Restored: Rhythm

This is not the end. It's the integration. The phase where everything steadies. You begin to live in flow with your days, your weeks, your seasons. You'll keep working, resting, and eating, but now, you do it in rhythm. Your rhythm. The one your body always remembered, but had forgotten how to follow, until now.

Phase 1
Build the Foundation

Length: ~ 4 weeks

Pillars Restored: Breath, Light, Water, Fire

We start here. Slow your breath. Feel the light. Let water move. It's a return to the things your body has always known.

Breathe Deep

Before anything else returns, the breath must.

There's a kind of breath you used to know, one that didn't rush or strain. It opened your chest without effort. It quieted your thoughts, steadied your nerves, and made space where tension used to live. But life got loud. Screens, stress, pressure. And the breath got shallow.

The Function

Breath is the body's original rhythm. It sets the tone for everything else - heart rate, nervous system, digestion, sleep, mood, focus. When the breath is tight or rushed, your body acts like it's under threat. But when your breath is deep and steady, your whole system gets the message, "it's safe."

Slow nasal breathing calms the nerves, improves oxygen delivery, and supports repair. It can help your body shift from alert to restore. Even a few minutes of steady breathing can create a full-body reset. This isn't 'breathwork'. It's your body remembering what steady feels like.

The Fracture

Most people were never taught how to breathe well. We sit in ways that collapse our ribs. We wear uncomfortable shoes that shift our natural posture. We spend hours talking or scrolling without ever noticing that we haven't taken a full breath. Tension builds. Our chest stiffens. Our breath shortens. And without realising it, we stop feeling relaxed in our own bodies.

The Return

- **Notice breath first |** Don't change it. Just observe. Spend time with one hand on your tummy, one on your chest. Learn your breath.
- **Breathe through your nose |** Mouth breathing bypasses your regulatory systems. Close your mouth when you're not speaking or eating. Some people find it beneficial to use mouth tape at night.
- **Pause before reacting |** One slow breath can interrupt a stress spiral. Use your breath to encourage calm, even in a busy world.
- **Sit or stand with open posture |** Create space at the ribs.
- **Breathe with movement |** Walk slowly outdoors and let your breath match your steps. Bring it back into rhythm.

Try a Breath Reset:

- Lie down with one hand on your belly, one on your chest.
- Let the breath reach the lower spine and lower ribs. Feel the tummy rise first.
- Inhale slowly through your nose for 4 seconds.
- Pause for a count of one.
- Exhale gently through your nose for 6 seconds. Then pause again.
- Don't worry about doing it perfectly. Just let the breath come back.
- Repeat for 5 - 10 minutes. Your body will relax and feel warm.

Signs of Restoration

You'll know it's working when something soft returns. Your shoulders drop, just a little. Your belly begins to soften, not by force, but by safety. You find yourself noticing your breath more often, and it begins to soothe you. You stop bracing. You start relaxing. And one day, you realise you're moving a little slower and with more presence.

Seasonal Shift

Spring | Breath may feel fast or shallow as your energy starts to rise. Use longer exhales to steady the change in season.

Summer | Breathing outdoors may feel energising. Mornings and evenings are great times to reset.

Autumn | As the air cools, you might notice tightness in the chest. Breathe slower. Let your breath create space.

Winter | Breath may feel slow or hidden. That's okay. Keep it gentle.

Let your breath be the first thing that returns.

Note | Help Along the Way

There's an appendix at the back with answers to common questions and a few extra tools to help along the way. Importantly, on page 216, "The Return Path" will guide you back to rhythm if you ever slip off track - whether from busyness, illness, or life itself. Feel free to flick there whenever you need. You don't have to read this book in a straight line.

And if at any point you need a little help choosing what to use - things like water filters, lamps, or electrolytes - you'll find a small collection of trusted resources at www.therhythmofhealth.com. Nothing pushy, just simple examples to help you begin and make the process feel easier.

Light that Charges

Receive light. Receive energy.

There's a certain kind of energy the body can only get from the sun. Not the gentle kind that wakes you in the morning, but a deeper charge, one that sinks through your skin and into your core. This is the moment the body refuels if you hold still long enough to receive. You feel it when you're stretched out on the grass, not thinking, just there. Warmth pressing into your bones. Breath soft. Muscles uncoiling. It's like your cells stop bracing. And something finally lands.

The Function

Midday full-spectrum sunlight helps the body receive energy. It's not about circadian rhythm just yet, it's about fuel. The melanin in your skin acts like tiny solar panels that collect and then transmit charge. The charge that fuels the mitochondria.

When paired with stillness or breath, the effect deepens. It can shift mood, relieve fatigue, and even help regulate appetite. For many people, this is the missing piece, the part that brings life back into the system.

This isn't about staying in the sun all day. It's about knowing your body, building a gentle tolerance, and using sunlight the way the body once did.

The Fracture

We moved indoors. We started fearing the sun, covering up completely, and working through the hours that used to be for rest and recharge. Many of us don't get full-spectrum sunlight at all anymore, only filtered light through glass. Over time, this drains the circuit. We lose the deep charge we were designed to receive. And the body starts showing signs. Tired eyes, flat mood, slow repair, unexplainable fatigue.

The Return

- **Get outside |** During the middle part of the day. Around 11 am to 2 pm, depending on your season.
- **Expose the skin |** Let your torso, back, arms, and legs receive light directly. No sunglasses, no hats. Start with a few minutes.
- **Lie down, don't stand |** When possible, lie on the ground. Let your body fully rest while charging. This slows the nervous system and creates a great environment to practise your breathing.
- **Turn over halfway |** Treat this like gentle sunbathing. Front, then back. You don't need a beach. A private backyard, a balcony, or a sunny patch of grass is enough.
- **Never burn |** Know your skin type and build exposure carefully and gradually. Trust your body's signals. If it starts to feel too much, then stop. Again, never burn.
- **Cool down after |** You may like to finish with a brief cold shower, especially if your body tends toward inflammation, histamine sensitivity, or leaky cell membranes. The cold helps calm the system, seal the cells, and lock in the charge.

Signs of Restoration

You'll know you're receiving light the way you once did when certain shifts begin to appear. You step outside and feel something lift. Your body begins craving stillness again, not distraction. The cold doesn't bite as sharply and warmth rises more easily. By mid-afternoon, you still feel steady, not drained. And one day, you catch your reflection and see it, the quiet glow returning to your skin.

Find Your Sunlight Starting Point

These times aren't strict rules, but starting points. They help you learn your skin's natural tolerance to the sun. But remember, sunlight isn't the same for everyone. Some medical conditions and medications can change how the body responds. If that's you, take care, and if you're unsure, check with your health professional.

Skin Type	Indicators	Starting Dose	Can Build Up To
Fair	Burns easily, rarely tans, often freckles. Light hair. Blue/green eyes.	3 - 5 minutes (front + back)	Up to 10 - 12 minutes (Stop at the first sign of pinkness)
Medium	Sometimes burns, usually tans after some sun. Brown/blonde hair. Brown/green eyes.	5 - 8 minutes (front + back)	Up to 15 - 20 minutes
Dark	High level of baseline pigment. Rarely burns, tans deeply. Dark hair. Dark brown eyes.	10 - 15 minutes (front + back)	Up to 20 - 40 minutes

Seasonal Shift

Spring | Start slow, your skin may be more sensitive after Winter. This is the time to build your solar base. Even short sessions make a difference.

Summer | Peak charge season. Get outside earlier or later in the day if the sun is strong. Prioritise full-body exposure without burning.

Autumn | Keep the habit going. The light is gentler but still powerful. This is a stabilising season, ideal for grounding alongside.

Winter | Even if you can't remove layers, still get outside. Face and hands count. Use brief sun breaks to top up your energy levels and lift mood.

Let light in. Then feel what rises.

First Hydrate

Drink what your cells can recognise.

Your body is made of water. But not just any water. It's the kind that flows, carries, responds, and remembers. The kind that knows how to move through you cleanly, quietly, and with direction. Somewhere along the way, you may have stopped drinking enough. Or started drinking the kind that doesn't really help. You didn't mean to. Life just got busy.

The Function

Water does more than hydrate. It carries signals. It carries charge. It carries minerals. It builds structure. It supports your brain, digestion, energy, fascia, joints, and circulation. When your body has the right kind of water (structured, mineralised, and flowing), your whole system starts working better. You think more clearly. You move more freely. Your skin feels more elastic. Your nervous system settles. This isn't about tracking litres. It's about remembering flow.

The Fracture

Most tap and bottled water today has been processed so heavily it no longer feels like water at all. Many modern sources are stripped, over-treated, or flavoured. Some even pull minerals out of your body.

At the same time, we over-caffeinate, under-hydrate, and forget to drink when we're actually thirsty. Over time, we lose charge and flow. The tissues stiffen. And the body quietly forgets how to absorb what it truly needs.

The Return

- **Start your morning with water |** Before coffee, before food. Try it with a pinch of sea salt. Let it wake and move the circuit.
- **Drink small amounts often |** This gives the body time and space to absorb what it receives.
- **Choose the best water you can |** Spring water is ideal. Filtered water that's been structured and re-mineralised with sea salt or trace mineral drops is also a great option. Choose the best water you can access *(See "How to Structure Water" on page 77).*
- **Choose still over sparkling, plain over flavoured |** Water closest to its most natural state is better recognised by the body.
- **Skip the plastic bottle |** Choose glass or stainless steel. It helps water hold its natural structure and stay pure.
- **Drink homemade bone broth |** This is one of the most effective ways to hydrate, remineralise, and nourish your cells. It's rich in sodium, potassium, collagen, amino acids, and deeply grounding. Just make sure it's homemade, as store-bought versions don't carry the same charge. *(There is a recipe in the appendix on page 227.)*

Signs of Restoration

You'll know hydration is working by how you feel. You wake with a little more alertness. Your joints feel less stuck and your body more fluid. Your skin softens, not from lotion, but from the inside. You find yourself reaching for water before you're told. You begin wanting clean water, structured water, and lose the pull toward drinks that used to mask thirst.

How to Structure Water

The way you treat your water changes how well your body can use it. When water flows in nature, over rocks, under sunlight, through earth, it picks up a natural structure. It becomes organised. Alive. Charged. But when it sits still in plastic or rushes through metal pipes, it loses that. It forgets how to flow.

Let it see light | Morning sunlight is best. Place a glass jug, filled with water, outside at sunrise. Light wakes water up, structures it, and fills it with charge.

Let it move | Pour it. Swirl it in a glass. Let it breathe. This simple swirling, sometimes called vortexing, reminds it how to flow.

Add a pinch of real salt | Not table salt, but salt with colour and minerals. You can also add a trace mineral drop if desired.

Most importantly, honour it. Don't just chug it distracted. Pause. Hold the glass. Breathe. Your intention matters more than you think.

Your digestion calms. Your mind steadies. And quietly, without fanfare, you feel more anchored.

Seasonal Shift

Spring | Your thirst may return suddenly, let your hydration rise with the light. Use the returning light to charge your water.
Summer | You may need more water and minerals than you think. Start early in the day and continue to sip throughout.

Autumn | Slow down your water intake as the light fades. Listen to your body's needs.

Winter | Your thirst might feel hidden. Drink warm or room temperature water to keep your system gently hydrated. Fresh homemade broth is great in Winter.

Not all water nourishes. Choose water that carries charge.

Supporting Water with Minerals

Your body doesn't just need water. It needs the minerals that help water land where it belongs, and stay there. Most people are running low on sodium, potassium, and magnesium without even knowing. You might feel foggy, flat, or drained. You might crave salt or wake up tired, even after sleep. Your joints might ache or you often cramp. These aren't failures, they're signals. Your body is asking for support.

Here's How to Begin

Sodium | Draws water into cells. Add a pinch of sea salt (like Celtic or Himalayan) to your water. Let your meals be salted to taste. Electrolytes and salt tablets can be used if you require more.

Potassium | Balances sodium and fluid. Found in many foods. You can use a supplement such as potassium citrate powder if more is needed.

Magnesium | Helps cells relax. Choose a gentle form like liquid magnesium pico-ionic formulas. It's rarer but worth seeking out. Most other forms absorb poorly. If new to magnesium, start small, build slowly.

Aim For

- **Sodium |** 4,000 - 6,000 mg / day (including from diet.)
- **Potassium |** 4,000 - 5,000 mg / day (including from diet.)
- **Magnesium |** 400 - 700 mg / (often in *addition* to diet.)

Note: Electrolyte needs vary. If you have a health condition or take medication that affects minerals, check in with your health professional.

... Continued

A Lived Example

One way to make this simple is to first track your food for a couple of days with a free app (like Cronometer). It gives you a sense of how much sodium and potassium you're already getting, and how much you may need to add.

- **Morning |** You start the day with a glass of water plus a pinch of sea salt. After breakfast, mix an electrolyte drink providing roughly 1,000mg sodium, 1,000mg potassium, and 200mg liquid magnesium.
- **Throughout the day |** Sip salted water to maintain hydration.
- **Evening |** Take a second electrolyte drink after dinner to top up.
- **On hot days or heavy work |** Sometimes a third glass of electrolytes might be added at lunch, to replace what was lost in sweat.

It doesn't have to be exact every day. Once you've got a sense of your baseline, it becomes intuitive. Some days your body asks for more, other days less. The goal isn't chasing numbers, it's learning to hear the signals. When the minerals are balanced, you feel clear, steady, and hydrated.

Listen to Your Body | If You Feel ...

- Dizzy, fatigued, foggy, low blood pressure, or crave salt → *add sodium.*
- Puffy, high blood pressure, or thirsty without relief → *reduce sodium.*
- Cramping, constipated, high heart rate, or flutters → *add potassium.*
- Weak, heavy, slow heart rate, or numbness → *reduce potassium.*
- Restless, tense, constipated, anxious, poor sleep → *add magnesium.*
- Nausea, diarrhoea, or stomach upset → *reduce magnesium.*

Let Movement Flow

Your body was never meant to hold still this long.

You weren't made to sit for hours or grind through routines that disconnect you. You were made to move like life itself - with breath, with joy, with rhythm. Your body was designed for walking, stretching, lifting, even dancing. When you move, even a little, something inside remembers how to soften. How to flow.

Movement isn't just for fitness. It's for life. It shifts the water in your tissues. It unwinds the fascia. It brings breath back to places you forgot were holding tight. This isn't about workouts. It's about waking up again.

The Function

Gentle movement keeps your body's waters flowing. When you move, even in simple ways, you create internal pressure that helps fluids reach every part of you. Your fascia stays hydrated and elastic. Joints glide. Breath returns.

Movement doesn't have to be intense to be effective. Gentle, spiral, wave-like motion unwinds stored compression, awakens proprioception, and helps the body find its orientation again. It clears stagnation. It loosens what's stuck. It creates just enough motion to remind your whole system that flow is still possible.

The Fracture

Most of us sit too long, stand too still, or move in rigid, repetitive ways. Chairs, screens, and concrete have replaced the rhythms we were built for. The result? Fascia dries out, and the body forgets how to move freely.

The Return

- **Walk every day |** The most powerful, overlooked movement there is. Let your feet touch the ground, let your breath match your stride.
- **Stretch what feels tight |** Follow sensation. Open your chest. Roll your spine. Let your limbs spiral. Let your body find new shapes.
- **Move slowly |** Let your nervous system feel each transition. Follow your breath. Move with intention.
- **Try rebounding or gentle bouncing |** Even a few minutes can clear your lymph and reawaken your fascia.
- **Release restrictions |** If tightness lingers, use a massage ball, foam roller, or skilled bodyworker to release tension and restore flow.
- **Use a standing desk |** Let your body re-learn how to shift, sway, and stay fluid while working.

Signs of Restoration

You'll know it's working when something inside you craves to move again. You start stretching without thinking. You catch yourself breathing deeper when you twist.

Your joints feel less stuck. You notice sensation in your limbs again. You feel lighter, like something finally let go. You feel fluid again, like water has found its way.

Seasonal Shift

Spring | Begin slowly, letting your body reawaken after the stillness of Winter. Use gentle movements - stretching, twisting, walking.

Summer | Move in the morning before the heat builds. Move freely. Let sweat and breath guide you. Open, expand, and enjoy movement.

Autumn | Shift toward steadier, grounding activity. Slow your rhythm, choosing movements that stabilise and connect you back to the earth.

Winter | Stay warm. Move to circulate. Don't push into exhaustion. Stretch the joints, fascia, spine. Rhythm over intensity.

Your body was made to move. Not just for fitness, but for flow.

Coming Up Next

At the end of each phase, you'll find a few tools to help bring the chapter to life. They're not instructions to follow word for word, but living examples, patterns you can lean on as you shape your own.

First, there's a *'Rhythm Checklist.'* A pared-back summary of the rhythms to work on, so you don't lose sight of the essentials.

Next, there's *'A Day in Rhythm.'* A simple outline of what life in rhythm might look like from sunrise to sleep. A way to picture how the pieces could weave together.

Finally, you'll see *'A Life in Rhythm'.* This is a short case study - a glimpse of what someone might notice when the principles of the phase take root.

Use these as guides. Borrow what resonates. Leave what doesn't. They're here to help you craft your own rhythm.

Phase 1 | Rhythm Checklist

This month is about laying down the foundations. Don't rush to master everything at once. Choose one, begin, then layer in the others as you feel ready. The monthly checklists are here to keep you anchored - a simple summary. Come back to it often, and re-read the chapter whenever you need more detail.

Breath

- ☐ Breathe through your nose whenever possible. Consider mouth taping.
- ☐ Practise the Breath Reset daily (4 - 1 - 6 - 1 nasal breathing).
- ☐ Match your breath with gentle movement - walking, stretching.

Light

- ☐ Get direct outdoor light on your skin most days.
- ☐ Building tolerance slowly. Know your skin type. Never burn.

Water

- ☐ Drink a glass of water first thing each morning with a pinch of salt.
- ☐ Choose clean water - spring or filtered. Sip steadily through the day.
- ☐ Structure your water with light, swirling and minerals.
- ☐ Work out your sodium, potassium, and magnesium needs, and start adding an electrolyte mix into your day.

Movement

- ☐ Walk outdoors every day, even briefly.
- ☐ Stretch, bounce, or twist the body to keep fascia and joints fluid.

Phase 1 | A Day in Rhythm

Morning

At sunrise, fill a glass jug with water and let it catch the first light. As the day begins, wake your body with a slow stretch. Open your chest, turn through your spine, breathe deep. Retrieve the jug with the water now charged with light. Add your minerals, swirl, and take it in. After breakfast, mix your first electrolyte drink. Sodium, potassium, magnesium. The day begins. Steady, charged, and clear.

Midday

Pause and meet the sun. A few minutes on your front, then on your back. Breathe slowly as you receive the light. Loosen again with a short stretch. Bends, twists, simple movements to wake your fascia and water again. Keep sipping clean, mineral-rich water through the day. On hotter days, take a small electrolyte top-up to keep the body charged.

Evening

After dinner, prepare one last electrolyte drink, then step outside for a walk. Let your breath fall into rhythm with your stride. When you return, settle with a cup of homemade bone broth, drinking slowly, mindfully. In bed, give yourself five minutes of gentle breath reset, softening the body toward sleep. If it feels right, try mouth taping at night to keep your breath calm and quiet.

A Life in Rhythm | James' Return to Hydration

James is 32 and works long days as a builder. He spends hours in the heat, sweating through his shirt by mid-morning. On weekends, he plays football, but lately the game hasn't felt the same. His stamina drops quickly, and his back has grown stiffer over the years. After a hamstring tear on the field, he came into clinic - not just for the injury, but because something deeper didn't feel right.

James drank plenty of water but never felt properly hydrated. His afternoons were a slog, his back ached, and stretching wasn't part of his routine. His body looked and felt tight, and he admitted he couldn't remember the last time he'd come close to touching his toes.

Over the next four weeks, James made small, steady changes. He added electrolytes to his water instead of drinking it plain. He began to twist and stretch gently each day, loosening the stiffness that had built up over years.

When he returned a month later, the difference was clear. His hamstring was healing well. His back no longer ached through the workday, and his energy didn't crash as hard in the afternoons. The moment that surprised him most - he could almost touch his toes, something he hadn't done in many years.

Phase 2
Reset the Body Clock

Length: ~ 4 weeks

Pillars Restored: Light, Fire, Rhythm

Time isn't the enemy. It's the rhythm your body longs to follow.

In this phase, light becomes your clock.

You'll wake, move, and rest at the right time, in the right way.

Let Light In

Let light reach you before anything else does.

There's a rhythm beneath everything. A rising and falling that holds the body in time. But somewhere along the way, most of us slipped out of sync. You may not even realise your rhythm is missing, only that you feel foggy, flat, or constantly behind.

The Function

Your body is designed to run on light. Not just for charge, but for timing. Morning light tells your body to wake up, to lift cortisol, to pause melatonin, and to open the gates to energy and movement. Midday light anchors the day, holding focus and energy steady. And evening light signals melatonin production and helps you wind down. These light signals are what keep your internal clock, your circadian rhythm, on track.

This rhythm aligns everything in your body, from your hormones to your heartbeat, from your digestion to your sleep. If the light doesn't reach you, the rhythm doesn't start. When it's aligned, the whole system runs like clockwork.

The Fracture

We wake up in darkness to alarms and miss the sun entirely. We live indoors, working under fluorescent lights. We scroll our phones late into the evening. The body no longer knows when it's time to rise, or when it's time to rest. The result? Hormones that are out of sync. Tired bodies. Restless minds. Poor sleep. And we don't realise that light is the missing puzzle piece.

The Return

- **Step outside within 30 minutes of waking |** No sunglasses. No screens. Watch the sunrise. Let natural light hit your eyes. This resets your internal clock and boosts energy.
- **Spend at least 20 minutes a day outdoors |** Your body needs full light exposure, not just filtered light through windows. Walk, stretch, or just sit outside.
- **Expose your skin to midday sun |** Even five minutes helps reinforce your natural rhythm *(see "Light That Charges" on page 71)*.
- **Watch the sunset |** This cues your system to slow down. Let your body see the light fade. Let it anchor your evenings.
- **Dim lights after dark |** Shift to warm, soft lighting in the evening. Avoid bright overheads and screens when possible. Consider using blue-blocking glasses with amber lenses if bright lighting is unavoidable.

Signs of Restoration

You'll feel it when the rhythm starts to return. You wake up before the alarm, not startled, but ready. Your day begins to move with rhythm, not resistance. Hunger and energy arrive early. Light feels good, not harsh. You crave it. Your mood steadies. Your mind clears. And at night, you sleep deeper. Like your body finally exhaled.

Seasonal Shift

Spring | Step outside early. Let morning light help your body adjust to longer days. Watch the light change.

Summer | Anchor your day in the full light. Use midday sun to keep your rhythm strong and battery charged.

Autumn | Light fades earlier as the days shorten. Let the sunset remind your system to settle. Wind down with it.

Winter | Rug up. Even dim light gives the signal. Light still reaches you, even through the cloud.

Let the sun set your clock.

Eat in Time

Before your body can heal, time must be restored.

Eating in rhythm is part of how the body knows it's time to heal and repair. Food isn't just about what you eat, but when. Your body isn't counting calories, but it is counting time. To eat out of rhythm is to confuse the system. To eat in rhythm is to return alignment.

By reducing your eating window, and by not eating late in the evening, your body receives the right signals about when to be active and when to rest. This means alert during the day. And relaxed at night. It also gives your body time to shift gears. Instead of just digesting all day, it starts repairing, detoxing, and healing.

The Function

Eating in rhythm with your body clock restores order. Your gut, liver, pancreas, and brain all run on daily cycles. They expect nourishment at certain windows, and rest and repair at others.

When food arrives on time, energy is used more efficiently. When food arrives late or constantly, energy becomes scattered and healing is stalled.

The Fracture

Modern eating has no clock. We graze all day, snack at night, feeding the body when it wants to clear. Your digestive system never gets a break. Your mitochondria stay stuck in "energy output" mode, and your body misses the opportunity to detox.

Bright lights delay our natural cues, and dinner has become later and later. We have forgotten when to eat. And it has dysregulated our sleep and wake hormones. Melatonin production is halted. Blood sugar and insulin rise at the wrong time. Leaving you wired but tired.

The Return

- **Anchor your first meal to the light |** Eat soon after the sun rises.
- **Keep your eating window short and consistent |** 8 - 10 hours between first and last bite is ideal.
- **Avoid eating late |** Aim to finish dinner at least 3 hours before bed. The earlier your last meal, the deeper the repair. Even small shifts can dramatically improve digestion and sleep.
- **Notice natural hunger |** Let your body tell you when it's ready, don't override it with routine. Not everyone needs three meals a day.
- **Avoid snacking |** Your digestive system needs breaks. If you feel you need to snack, try having a bigger, more nourishing breakfast.
- **Match food types to timing |** Heartier in the morning, lighter in the evening. It matches fuel to when your body can use it best.

Signs of Restoration

You'll know it's working when rhythm starts to guide your eating instead of rules. Hunger returns at consistent times. You fall asleep faster, and sleep runs deeper. Your digestion quiets. Bloating fades. And you crave earlier meals and lighter evenings.

If You're Wondering | "Is This Even Working?"

Healing doesn't always shout. Sometimes it whispers. You might not lose all your symptoms in the first week. You might not feel clear, light, or energised right away. Sometimes the body gets quiet. Or tired. Or unsure. That doesn't mean you're failing. It means something is shifting underneath.

Keep going. Rest more. Trust the rhythm. Let the body rebuild before you judge the result. Not all change is loud.

Seasonal Shift

Spring | Your digestion may be slower after Winter. Choose warm, easy-to-digest foods in the morning.
Summer | Longer light means slightly extended eating windows feel natural, but still finish a few hours before bed.
Autumn | Begin to shorten the eating window again. Let grounding meals support slowing energy.
Winter | Eat with intention. Use warm broths, hearty stews, and early dinners to align with the season.

Let meals follow daylight. Let nights be empty.

Return to Dark

Light ends the day, but darkness seals it.

There's a softness that comes with the end of the day. It's not loud. It doesn't push. It's the kind of quiet that tells your body to let go. Muscles stop bracing. Eyes grow heavy. You feel it when the sun dips low and the light turns gold. Your system knows, it's time to wind down.

But we've replaced it with scrolling. Blue light. Noise. We've made the night feel like midday. And your body doesn't know how to land. To heal, you must return to dark. It's what tells your body, "you're safe now."

The Function

As the sun sets, light slows down. Wavelengths stretch out to amber, gold, and red. That shift signals the body to return. You move from output to restoration. Cortisol drops. Melatonin rises. Your nervous system receives the cue that it's safe to stop. And when you honour it, your system softens before you even lie down. Breath deepens. Muscles release. And repair begins before the day is done.

The Fracture

Most of us never see the sunset anymore. We go from high-speed days into bright rooms and blue-lit nights. These artificial lights mimic the midday sun and confuse the brain. So instead of slowing down, your system stays alert. Your body doesn't get the message, "rest now." Sleep feels harder. You wake up still tired because recovery is delayed.

The Return

- **Step outside around sunset |** Even five minutes cues the body.
- **Dim the lights as evening begins |** Use globes with warm tones like amber, red, and gold.
- **Use candles and salt lamps |** For soft grounding light.
- **Shift your screen settings |** After sunset, use warmer tones to ease your body into night. Simple, free apps can help with this.
- **Let sound quiet |** No fast talking or loud music. Let sound follow the dark. Gentle music or the crackling of a fire to slow the body.
- **Set a tech-off time |** 8pm or earlier. Switch to books, journaling, music, and quiet conversation. Let your body settle.
- **Wear amber blue-blocking glasses |** If you can't avoid screens at night, amber lenses help filter the blue light.

Signs of Restoration

As you return to dark, you begin to feel the difference in your body. You no longer push through the evening, instead, you feel yourself naturally drawn into rest. Your thoughts slow down after dinner. There's a stillness that enters, and it feels good. The restlessness fades. Instead of pacing or reaching for stimulation, you find yourself wanting quiet. Wanting soft. Wanting slow. The body isn't fighting the night anymore. It's following it.

Seasonal Shift

Spring | Step outside at dusk. Let shifting light reset your rhythm, and remind your body it's time to wind down.

Summer | Use the long twilight. Dim lights slowly. Let your body taper with the light. If darkness comes too late, wear amber lens blue-blocking glasses about two hours before bed to help signal sleep.

Autumn | Darkness arrives sooner. Honour it. Let quiet come early. Observe the light change.

Winter | Embrace the dark. Keep lights low. Stretch the stillness. Your circuit needs the deep repair that Winter brings.

Descent is not collapse. Let the night speak again.

When Your Body Doesn't Feel Safe

Sometimes, you try to rest, but your body won't let you. You try to eat well, but your digestion won't have it. You try to slow down, but your mind won't quiet. You're not failing. And you're not broken. Your nervous system is trying to protect you.

It runs on two modes. One is the alert system (sympathetic), and it gets you ready to fix, act, defend. The other is the restore system (parasympathetic), and it's where healing, digestion, detox and repair happen.

If your body doesn't feel safe, it can't shift into restore mode, no matter how many health changes you try. This is why rhythm sometimes doesn't land at first. Your system might need more quiet. More time. More proof that the pressure is gone. You don't have to force that shift. Simply invite it. And each time you return, your body learns what safety feels like.

To move from alert to restore, try this:
- **Slow your breath** | Exhale longer than you inhale.
- **Add a soft pause** | After you exhale, rest 1 - 3 seconds before the next inhale. With practice, lengthen to 5 - 8 second pauses.
- **Try progressive muscle relaxation** | Helps relax the body from head to toe. Many simple guided versions are available online.
- **Talk it through** | A good counsellor can help uncover and release stress that keeps your system stuck in alert mode.
- **Put bare feet on the ground** | Just one minute can reset the body.
- **Listen to something calm** | Gentle sounds relax and restore.
- **Place a hand on your chest or belly** | Say softly, "*You're safe now.*"

Sleep Deep

This is where the body returns, to rebuild, to heal.

You don't sleep by trying. You sleep when the body feels safe. Sleep is not a task. It's not something you win or fail at. It's a consequence of alignment.

If the day was ordered, if the cues were honoured, sleep arrives. If not, no amount of supplements, darkness, or silence can force it. Sleep isn't earned. It's allowed.

When sleep is off, everything feels heavier. Not just tired, but scattered. Like you've been leaking energy without noticing. But when sleep is strong, the system heals. Hunger calms. Emotions settle. Energy returns.

The Function

Seeing sleep as a response, not a goal, shifts everything. You don't need to chase it. You remove what blocks it. Sleep becomes your nightly audit, not of how hard you tried, but of how well you lived in rhythm.

Sleep is the deepest layer of repair. The brain clears waste. Tissues mend. Stress drains from the nervous system. Hormones reset. Sleep holds rhythm together. When sleep is strong - appetite, focus, mood, and tolerance rise. When it's weak - everything slips.

The Fracture

Modern life chips away at sleep without meaning to. Screens. Late food. Overthinking. Shallow breath. Constant noise. We lost rhythm, then blamed ourselves for not "switching off."

But sleep doesn't obey willpower. It listens for signals. And when those signals vanish, so does the depth. Over time, we forget how to drop in. Sleep becomes shallow. Mornings feel heavy. And tired becomes normal.

The Return

- **Stop solving sleep** | It's not a project. Rhythm matters more.
- **Wake with the sun** | Timing is more important than total hours. Wake to see the morning light to anchor your circadian rhythm.
- **Avoid caffeine after 2pm** | Even if you fall asleep, it can still disrupt the quality of your rest. Lighter sleep, and less repair.
- **Finish eating at least 3 hours before bed** | Digestion competes with deep sleep by blocking melatonin production.
- **Dim the lights 1 - 2 hours before bed** | Softer light helps your body release melatonin. Amber glasses help if screens are hard to avoid.
- **Keep phones out of the bedroom** | Or use airplane mode to keep your bedroom quiet and restful. Switch off Wi-Fi if possible.
- **Block all light while sleeping** | Even small amounts confuse your body. Use a sleep mask if necessary.
- **Early to bed** | The deepest repair happens in the first hours of sleep, roughly between 10pm and 2am for most people.
- **Keep the room cool (16 - 19°C)** | A drop in body temperature cues sleep, and a cooler room helps that happen.
- **Use natural, breathable bedding** | Cotton, wool, linen. Your body needs to regulate temperature and natural bedding helps.
- **Make bedtime a ritual** | Simple. Quiet. Repeated. Your body learns through pattern and rhythm.

Signs of Restoration

Sleep begins to return when the striving stops. You fall asleep without needing to scroll. You wake without that heavy fog. Your mornings feel lighter. Your cravings soften, no longer reaching for sugar or caffeine just to get through. And instead of feeling flat or depleted, you begin to feel restored. Not just rested.

Seasonal Shift

Spring | Let mornings be bright. Wake with the sun, open the windows, and let early light draw you out of sleep. Nights can still hold depth.

Summer | Longer days can delay rest. Dim the lights early. Use amber lens glasses 1 - 2 hours before bed. Cooler bedding and airflow matter.

Autumn | Let evenings lengthen. Begin dimming the lights earlier. Sleep grows deeper when you match the darker nights.

Winter | Honour the long nights. Extra sleep is not laziness - it's repair. Let your body lean into rest. The body longs for deep healing.

Sleep comes when the body feels safe to let go.

What About Shift Work?

Shift work goes against the grain of our biology. Our hormones, mitochondria, and nervous system, were all designed to follow the rhythm of light and dark.

When that rhythm flips, night becomes day, meals are in the dark, sleep is during the light, the body struggles. Not because it's weak, but because it's ancient. It remembers what time is. And artificial timing creates confusion. We see the effects:

- Poor sleep, chronic fatigue, brain fog.
- Higher rates of heart disease, diabetes, mood disorders.
- Disrupted hormones, weight gain.
- Weakened mitochondria, slowed healing.

But this isn't about shame. Many people work nights to serve others, to provide, to care. It's needed. So what can be done?

If You Work Shifts, Here's What Might Help

- **Prioritise "morning" light (when you wake) |** Even if it's 4pm, go outside. Let the light hit your eyes. This resets your inner clock.
- **Use darkness strategically |** On night shifts, dim artificial lights when possible. Avoid bright blue lights near the end of shift. Wear blue-blocking glasses. Protect the signal of "night."
- **After your shift, recreate sundown |** As you wind down, avoid screens, bright LEDs. Use warm lamps. Amber lens glasses. Tell your body it's bedtime.

... Continued

- **Sleep in a cave** | Use blackout curtains, eye masks, earplugs. Your sleep needs to be deep, even if it's during the day.
- **Support your mitochondria** | Eat real food, avoid sugar (Phase 5). Replenish minerals. Use cold exposure when you can (Phase 4). Your cells are working harder to make up for the disrupted rhythm.
- **Anchor to something stable** | Find a non-negotiable rhythm, a steady routine. Breath practice. Morning grounding. A quiet stretch. Something that happens at the same time every day, no matter your shift. This becomes your body's compass.

This is not perfect. The circadian clock still suffers. But these tools help reduce the damage, anchor the body, and keep some internal order alive. And when the season shifts, when the time comes to return to light and to rhythm, the body will remember.

Phase 2 | Rhythm Checklist

This month is about resetting the body clock. Don't try to overhaul everything overnight. Begin with light, then layer in rhythm around meals, and sleep.

Light

- ☐ Step outside within 30 minutes of waking and watch the sunrise.
- ☐ Head outside at intervals through the day to receive natural light.
- ☐ Watch the sunset or step outside at dusk to help align your body clock.
- ☐ Dim lights after dark. Use warm lamps and candles to signal evening.

Meals

- ☐ Anchor your first meal to the morning light.
- ☐ Keep meals within an 8 - 10 hour window and avoid snacking between.
- ☐ Finish eating at least three hours before bed so melatonin can rise.
- ☐ Choose heartier meals earlier, lighter meals later.

Sleep

- ☐ Avoid caffeine after 2pm to protect sleep.
- ☐ Set a tech-off time (ideally 8pm or earlier).
- ☐ Keep your room dark, cool (16 - 19°C), and free of phones and Wi-Fi.
- ☐ Aim to fall asleep before 10 pm for deepest repair.
- ☐ Build a simple bedtime ritual, your body learns through pattern.

Phase 2 | A Day in Rhythm

Morning

At sunrise, fill a glass jug with water and let it catch the first light. Step outside, stretch gently, and watch the day begin. When you return, drink water structured by light, with minerals stirred in. Sit down to a hearty meal, solid fuel to carry you through the day. Then mix your first electrolyte drink. Begin steady and charged.

Midday

Pause and meet the sun. Several minutes on your front, then your back. Let your body loosen with a short stretch to wake your fascia and move the water. Sit to a full lunch, enough to steady you so snacks aren't needed. Keep sipping water through the afternoon, clean, mineral-rich, unhurried.

Evening

Eat an early, light dinner, finished well before bedtime. Afterward, take your final electrolyte drink and step out for a walk at sunset, watching the light fade. When you return, dim the lights, soften the sound, switch off the tech. Let the house settle into quiet. Reading, gentle conversation, nothing that pulls you out of rhythm. Close the evening with a cup of broth, sealing the day. At night, give yourself five minutes to reset your breath. Let it soften you into sleep.

A Life in Rhythm | Johnny's Reset

Johnny is 38 and spends most of his time in an office. He's ambitious, driven, and always connected. Screens glow from morning until late into the night, emails keep him wired, and sleep feels like something he never quite reaches. By the time he came into clinic, he was plagued with headaches and admitted that even when he felt exhausted, he couldn't switch off enough to sleep deeply.

Johnny's body clock was out of rhythm. Meals were scattered, daylight was scarce, and his work blurred into the night. The more he pushed, the less efficient he became.

Over the next few weeks, Johnny made deliberate shifts. He started eating his main meals earlier, in line with daylight. He built in short outdoor breaks, just enough to remind his body what time it was. In the evenings, he dimmed the lights, set screens aside earlier, and sometimes used amber glasses if he had to finish a task.

The change was gradual but steady. His sleep began to deepen. His headaches eased. And with better rest came sharper focus during the day. He found himself getting more done without dragging his nights into overtime. What surprised him most was the sense of space - time in the evenings to breathe, to sit quietly, even to enjoy the dark rather than resist it.

Phase 3
The Right Environment

Length: ~ 4 weeks

Pillars Restored: Breath, Land

Your body heals best in safety.
When the air is clean, the ground is near, and your space feels like peace.
This phase clears the noise so the body can land.

Clean the Air

Let your breath land in safety.

There's something your body does without you even noticing. It breathes. It pulls in what's around you and carries it deep into your system, straight to your blood, your brain, your cells. So if the air around you is full of dust, mould, chemicals, or synthetic scents, then that's what your body takes in. And if the air doesn't feel safe, your body doesn't feel safe either.

You might not notice it straight away. Just a tightness. A fog. Maybe you're always tired, or your chest feels heavy indoors. Maybe your sinuses stay blocked or your immune system stays stuck in high alert. You're not just reacting to life, you're reacting to the air. Let the air around you match what your breath desires.

The Function

Clean air gives your nervous system permission to relax. It lets your immune system stand down. It gives your breath somewhere to land without resistance. Your lungs are not filters. So when you breathe in mould spores, dust particles, smoke, synthetic fragrances, or cleaning fumes, your body has to deal with all of it. That can trigger irritation, inflammation, allergic reactions, even chronic fatigue.

When the air is clean, your breath becomes fuel. Your oxygen uptake improves. Your focus sharpens. Your immune system calms. Your whole body begins to feel like it can exhale.

The Fracture

We sealed our buildings to keep out the weather, but trapped stale air inside. We sprayed artificial scents to mask odours, but coated our lungs in perfume. We filled rooms with plastic, vinyl, foam, and synthetics, all of which release chemicals into the air, even years after they're made.

Then came the mould. From damp corners, old carpets, leaky roofs, unventilated bathrooms. Invisible but potent. And now, many of us are breathing air that was never meant to be inside us. Our bodies weren't made to live in sealed boxes. We need fresh air. Real air.

The Return

- **Open windows daily** | Even for ten minutes. Let new air in.
- **Check for mould** | Behind furniture, under sinks, around showers. If you smell must or see black-green specks, take action.
- **Clove oil for mould** | Wipe visible mould with a mix of vinegar and a few drops of clove oil. One of the most effective ways to kill it at the source. You'll find a simple recipe at www.therhythmofhealth.com.
- **Diffuse clove oil** | A few drops in a bedside mist diffuser can support recovery if you've been reacting to mould.
- **Rinse your sinuses** | If you are affected by dust, mould or pollen, or work in a dusty environment, rinsing once or twice a day with saline solution helps clear irritants and calm the airways.
- **Bring in plants** | Indoor plants act as natural filters, pulling toxins from the air while adding oxygen and moisture.
- **Avoid synthetic scents** | Skip air fresheners, perfumes, chemical candles and fragrance in cleaning products.

- **Switch to natural cleaners |** Vinegar, bicarb, essential oils, or unscented options. They work just as well.
- **Vacuum and mop often |** Dust builds up fast, especially in corners and under furniture.
- **Wipe surfaces regularly |** Including window frames, fans, vents.
- **Choose natural materials |** Cotton, wood, wool, glass, over plastic, synthetic, and foam. Off-gassing drops when you simplify.
- **Use an air purifier |** Especially if you live in a city or can't open the windows often.
- **Use a dehumidifier |** In damp climates or poorly ventilated homes, a dehumidifier can dry the air and help discourage mould growth.

Signs of Restoration

When your air clears, your breath deepens. Your head feels lighter. That strange pressure in your sinuses eases. You cough less. Your chest stops bracing. Even your skin can calm. You might not notice it all at once. But quietly your body starts to trust the air again.

Seasonal Shift

Spring | Check for mould after Winter. Clean fans, vents, windows. Open up the house and let new air in.
Summer | Let air flow through. Be sure to keep humidity in check.
Autumn | Watch for hidden damp. Wipe window condensation. Stay alert to musty smells.
Winter | Air the house when the sun's out. Even cold air is better than stale air. Let your space breathe.

Let your air be clean enough to trust.

Honour the Surface

What you touch, touches back.

Every day, your skin meets the world. Bedsheets. Clothes. Floors. Sofas. Chairs. Your hands, your face, your whole body, constantly brushing against something. But what you touch doesn't just sit on the surface. It speaks to your nervous system. It speaks to your body. It either helps you soften and breathe, or it keeps your body on alert. Braced. Compressed.

We were meant to live in contact with living things. Wood. Wool. Cotton. Clay. Stone. Linen. Earth. But over time, we replaced those with plastic, foam, polyester, vinyl, and chemically treated fabrics. And the body feels the difference even if the mind doesn't know why.

The Function

Natural surfaces calm the body. They breathe. They let your skin relax. They help your nervous system drop down a gear. And because your skin and fascia are full of sensory receptors, the message is instant, "this is safe."

Synthetic surfaces on the other hand often trap heat, block breath, hold static, or off-gas chemicals. Over time, that can lead to irritation, sleep issues, restlessness, even vague fatigue that's hard to trace. Your body doesn't want to be on high alert. It wants to exhale.

The Fracture

We stopped noticing. We bought what looked nice, what was cheap, or what was trending. We filled our homes with fast furniture, foam mattresses, polyester bedding, plastic flooring. Then we wondered why we felt wired in our own homes. Why our sleep felt shallow. Why our skin itched. Why we couldn't fully settle. It wasn't just stress. It was contact. And slowly, our systems stopped feeling safe.

The Return

- **Switch to natural bedding |** Try cotton, wool, or linen bedding. It allows your body to breathe and rest more easily.
- **Use a wool pillow |** Breathable, supportive, and naturally resistant to dust mites and mould. Many companies now offer woollen pillows and even mattresses.
- **Choose breathable fabrics for clothing |** Cotton, hemp, bamboo, linen, or wool over polyester or synthetics.
- **Check your mattress |** If it's made from foam, consider a natural woollen topper as a buffer layer. It will also help your body to regulate temperature.
- **Lay down a natural rug or mat |** Jute, hemp, or wool rugs help ground your space and bring warmth without synthetic fibres.
- **Minimise synthetics where you sit |** Even a simple cotton throw or lambskin over a chair can soften the contact.
- **Choose personal products with care |** What touches your skin enters your body. Make-up, cleansers, moisturisers, toothpastes, deodorants, shampoos - all send signals through the surface. Keep them simple, with ingredients your body knows. Consider tallow or clay-based products.

Signs of Restoration

When surfaces change, your body softens. You feel less braced. Your skin breathes. You sit longer without fidgeting. You don't toss and turn as much. You wake up more rested, even if nothing else changed.

Seasonal Shift

Spring | Wash bedding and air it outside. Let natural fibres breathe.

Summer | Lighter layers. Natural fabrics help the skin cool and wick away sweat without trapping heat.

Autumn | Transition to warmth. Add wool or cotton throws instead of synthetic fleece.

Winter | Layer in grounding textures. Choose fibres that insulate and breathe like wool. Your body will settle better.

Let your skin touch what makes it feel safe.

Make Room to Breathe

Your home holds your nervous system.

Most of us don't realise how loud our homes have become, not with sound, but with stuff. Shelves packed. Counters crowded. Closets overflowing. Every room asking something of us. Move this. Clean that. Fix this. Finish that. And when your eyes never land on stillness, your body doesn't either.

The nervous system takes in everything you see, even what you've stopped noticing. And when your space is full, so is your mind. But stillness can return. Not by throwing everything out. Not by chasing minimalism. But by making space for peace again.

The Function

Creating open space helps the nervous system reset. It lets light move. It lets breath deepen. It tells your body there's nothing to do right now. You can soften here.

Even one clear corner changes the tone of a whole room. A small bench by the window. A bare spot on the floor with a cushion. A space with nothing to fix, nothing to store. It lets your body know that it's safe to rest here.

The Fracture

We got fast. We filled our carts. We bought on impulse, on sale, on emotion. We filled every shelf, every drawer, every surface. We made homes that stimulate, not soothe.

The result? Rooms that feel heavy. No space to exhale. No clear zone to land. And instead of peace, our homes became projects. Instead of rest, we feel tension. Stillness didn't leave us. We covered it.

The Return

- **Clear one spot |** A corner, a bench, a ledge. Let it be simple. Nothing on it. Nothing around it. Just space.
- **Pause before buying |** When you feel the urge to get something new, ask: "Do I need more? Or do I need stillness instead?"
- **Let light return |** Open curtains. Clean windows. Let light hit bare surfaces. Natural light softens a room and helps it feel alive again.
- **Create a still spot |** A chair by a window, a mat on the floor, a cushion on the porch. A place you can sit for five minutes without a goal.
- **Keep surfaces simple |** One bowl, one book, one lamp. Empty space is not waste. It's breath.
- **Walk through your home slowly |** If you feel tension, clutter, or compression in a room, try removing just one thing. Notice what changes.

Signs of Restoration

You'll feel your space shift before you see it. You'll walk into a room and exhale without knowing why. Your mind will quiet just by sitting down. You'll stop filling silence with screens. You'll crave fewer things. You'll reach for slowness, not distraction.

Seasonal Shift

Spring | Open the windows. Clear a corner. Let light touch surfaces again.

Summer | Keep surfaces light. Too much around you feels heavy in the heat. Space brings ease. Lighten the load.

Autumn | Slow the inputs. Choose what stays, choose what goes. Make room for grounding textures. Let rooms hold only what steadies you.

Winter | Create room for rest. A still chair, an uncluttered corner. A place to sit quietly in the darker months.

Make space that doesn't ask anything of you.
Let your home breathe so your body can too.

Ground the Body

You were never meant to live unplugged.

Electricity only works if it has somewhere to return. That's why every circuit has a ground, a point of contact that completes the loop. Without it, charge builds up. Systems short out. Energy can't settle. Your body is no different.

You are an electrical system. Light, breath, movement, thought - every signal your body sends runs on charge. But if there's nowhere for that charge to go, it builds. It scatters. It leaks. That's what grounding is. Not a wellness trend. Not something to buy. It's simply returning the body to contact. Real contact with the earth.

The Function

When your skin touches the ground, bare feet on soil, hands in the garden, lying on grass, your body begins to regulate. Static discharges. Inflammation eases. The nervous system can shift.

This happens through electrons - tiny, negatively charged particles the earth holds in abundance. When you touch the earth directly, those electrons flow into you and neutralise excess positive charge in your system from stress and inflammation. It's physics. It's simple. It's real. You don't need to understand every mechanism. You'll feel it. A softening. A slowing. A weight dropping down through your bones. That's the circuit completing.

The Fracture

We covered our feet in rubber and plastic. We built houses off the ground. We lived upstairs, worked indoors, and walked on sealed concrete. We made sure nothing we touched was real. And now, our bodies are full of charge with nowhere to send it. Our sleep is shallow. Our minds are fast. And our nervous systems are stuck in the "on" position. We disconnected from the very thing that stabilises us.

The Return

- **Stand barefoot on real ground |** Dirt, grass, sand, stone. If barefoot isn't possible, grounding sandals work too - they let charge flow while protecting your feet.
- **Lie down on the earth |** Stretch out. Breathe. Let your spine and skin make contact. Even five minutes can shift something deep.
- **Use your hands |** In the garden. In the sand. Your palms conduct too. Give them something real to hold.
- **Be consistent |** The effect builds. Even short, frequent moments add up. Each time you touch the ground, your system settles a little more.

What About Grounding Tools?

Some people use grounding mats or pads. They can give a hint of connection, but they're not the same as the earth itself. Don't let gear replace what's free. The point isn't to buy connection. The point is to return to it.

Signs of Restoration

You'll know grounding is working when the noise in your head quiets. When your breath drops deeper without effort. When you feel heavier, in a good way. Your sleep may deepen. Pain may ease. You begin to crave the ground itself, not out of theory, but from your body knowing this is right.

Seasonal Shift

Spring | Let bare feet return. Walk slowly. Let the earth feel you again.

Summer | Lie on grass. Sit on rocks. Stretch in the sand. Let charge release.

Autumn | Stay connected even as it cools. Grounding helps prepare the body for the quieter seasons.

Winter | Ground through hands. Natural floors. Skin contact still matters. Cold is not the enemy, disconnection is.

You were never meant to carry it all.
Let the ground receive what your body cannot hold.

Restore the Gut

Your gut is where the outside enters in.

Your gut isn't just a place where food gets digested. It's home to trillions of tiny organisms, bacteria, fungi, and microbes that make up what's called your microbiome.

This inner ecosystem affects almost everything. How you digest food, how strong your immune system is, how steady your energy feels, even how your brain functions. But for many people, that balance has been thrown off. It's called dysbiosis. When the helpful microbes are reduced and the unhelpful ones take over, the gut is thrown out of balance - and so is the rest of you.

The Function

When your microbiome is healthy, digestion flows more smoothly. Bloating reduces. Your immune system calms down. Nutrients get absorbed. Your energy feels more stable. Even your mood can lift.

That's because the microbes in your gut help you process food, make vitamins, manage inflammation, and send messages to the brain through the gut-brain axis. They're not just passengers. They're active helpers.

Restoring that balance means creating an environment where the helpful microbes can grow and the unhelpful ones can't take over.

The Fracture

Years of processed foods, antibiotics, low-quality diets, chronic stress, and environmental toxins have damaged many people's gut microbiomes, often without them realising.

But it's not just the obvious things. Constant snacking keeps the gut too busy to clean itself. Lack of outdoor exposure means we miss the microbes our bodies used to receive from soil, plants, and animals. We use antibacterial sprays and wipes. We rely on sugar and refined starches to get through the day. Many people live with hidden food intolerances they've never identified. And underneath it all, low stomach acid or long-term gut inflammation quietly disrupt digestion.

Most people don't connect their gut to their symptoms. They just feel tired. Foggy. Bloated. Inflamed. Like nothing is working. But often, the real problem lives in their microbiome.

The Return

- **Eat whole, unprocessed foods |** Meals made from real ingredients feed the good bacteria in your gut and help them grow.
- **Cut back on sugar and processed starches |** These feed harmful bacteria and yeast, crowding out the ones that keep you well.
- **Eat slower, chew well |** Digestion starts in the mouth. Don't rush.
- **Drink lightly with meals |** Small sips are fine, but avoid large amounts of fluid while eating or soon after. Too much liquid can dilute stomach acid and rush food through the gut before it's ready.
- **Support Digestion |** Apple cider vinegar or a broad digestive enzyme before meals can help your body break food down more easily.
- **Include broths and warm, soft foods |** They support digestion and help soothe and repair the gut lining.
- **Avoid constant snacking |** Your gut needs breaks to clean itself.

- **Spend time outdoors** | Exposure to soil, plants, and animals helps reintroduce healthy microbes.
- **Reduce stress** | Stress changes the gut environment and slows repair. Even five minutes of deep breathing can reset the circuit.

When Rhythm Isn't Enough

For many people, restoring rhythm is enough to see change. But for others, the gut has deeper layers of imbalance.

If your microbiome is overgrown by bacteria in the wrong place (SIBO), fungi like Candida, or parasites, you might feel like you're doing everything right and still not getting better. That doesn't mean you've failed. It just means your gut needs a little more support.

Possible signs of internal overgrowth include:
- Intense sugar or carb cravings that feel hard to control.
- Bloating after meals, especially with fibre or carbs.
- A coated tongue or strange body odour.
- Fatigue that hits shortly after eating.
- Brain fog or mood swings with no clear cause.
- Skin flares, rashes, or itchiness without a known trigger.

These issues are more common than you think. If you've already been following the rhythm practices in this book but feel like you've stalled, turn to the appendix: "When You've Tried Everything and Still Feel Stuck." That section will guide you toward deeper steps, so your body can clear what's standing in the way.

Signs of Restoration

When your microbiome begins to heal, your body quiets. Your bloating reduces. Your mood steadies. Your skin changes. You stop reacting to every food. Even your cravings shift. You don't just digest better. You feel calmer in your body.

Seasonal Shift

Spring | Reintroduce fresh, lighter foods, but go gently. After Winter, the gut may be more sensitive, so small steps help it adjust.
Summer | Keep meals light and simple. Spend time outdoors, eat close to nature, and let food diversity return.
Autumn | Slow it down. Focus on warm, simple meals that ground you as the days shorten.
Winter | Lean into broths, stews, and comfort meals. Eat foods that are soft and easy to digest.

Your gut needs rhythm, patience, and a little space to return.

Phase 3 | Rhythm Checklist

This month is about creating safety. Clean air. Calm space. Real ground. Steady gut. Start with one area and make changes gradually.

Home & Surfaces

- ☐ Open windows daily for 10 - 20 minutes. Cross-ventilate if possible.
- ☐ Let natural light in by opening curtains and cleaning windows.
- ☐ Hunt for damp and mould and address early.
- ☐ Choose simple cleaners - vinegar, bicarb, essential oils.
- ☐ Keep dust low with regular cleaning, vacuuming and wiping.
- ☐ Clear clutter and create one still corner in each room.
- ☐ Favour cotton, linen, bamboo and wool for everyday clothing.
- ☐ Switch to natural bedding - cotton, linen, wool.
- ☐ Choose natural personal care products.

Grounding

- ☐ Bare feet on real earth for five minutes daily.
- ☐ Combine with breath or gentle sunbathing for a deeper reset.
- ☐ If the ground is rough or cold, use grounding sandals.

Gut

- ☐ Choose wholefoods and reduce sugar and refined products.
- ☐ Take three calm breaths before eating and chew slowly.
- ☐ Consider a teaspoon of apple cider vinegar in water before meals.
- ☐ Avoid large amounts of fluid during or right after meals.

Phase 3 | A Day in Rhythm

Morning

At sunrise, set out your water to charge in the light. Step outside barefoot, stretch while the sun lifts over the horizon. When you return, drink mineral-rich, structured water. Sit to a hearty breakfast of whole, unprocessed food, eaten slowly. Mix a glass of electrolytes and sip it through the morning. Choose natural fabrics for your clothing. Use simple, clean skincare. Make the bed, tidy a corner, open the windows. These small resets hold the day steady.

Midday

Pause and meet the sun. Several minutes on your front, then your back, grounding if you can. Loosen your body with a short stretch. Sit down to lunch. Nourishing, unprocessed food, eaten without rush. No snacks needed as the meal carries you steady. Keep the rhythm of water through the day, mineral-rich and clean.

Evening

Eat an early, light dinner. Drink electrolytes. Step out for a sunset walk, barefoot if you can, watching the light fade. When you return, dim the lights, quiet the sound, switch off the tech. Let the house soften. Settle with a cup of broth and reading in a favourite chair, in a space that feels restful and safe. The bedroom is cool and dark, with natural bedding that lets the body breathe. In bed, follow your breath, let it calm you.

A Life in Rhythm | Nicole's Shift

Nicole is 43 and splits her time between admin work and caring for her kids. For years she's struggled with blocked sinuses, puffiness around her eyes, and occasional skin flares that never seemed to fully settle. Nothing serious on paper, but enough to make her feel drained and uncomfortable. She came into clinic hoping for relief.

A few questions revealed that her symptoms often flared at home. Moisture was hard to manage in the house, with mould creeping onto bathroom tiles, bedroom windows, even spots inside the washing machine. She admitted she'd learned to live with it, relying on the odd antihistamine, but never really tackling the source.

Nicole decided to change her environment instead of just chasing symptoms. She swapped her pillows for natural wool ones, resistant to dust mites. She gave the house a deep clean, cleared the mould, tidied clutter, and invested in a dehumidifier to keep the dampness down. She also began rinsing her sinuses each evening to clear irritants before bed.

The changes weren't instant, but over time her body began to calm. Her sinuses opened more easily, her skin reacted less, and she noticed she didn't wake up as foggy or congested.

Nicole's story showed her what many overlook - the body doesn't just respond to food or medicine - it responds to the air, the surfaces, and the spaces we live in.

Phase 4
Build Your Mitochondria

Length: ~ 4 - 6 weeks

Pillars Restored: Breath, Light, Fire

You're not fragile - your cells know how to fire.
Here, you'll build the signals that ignite strength from within.
Gentle challenges, cold, and light that rebuilds.

Embrace the Cold

Let the cold teach your body how to burn.

Your body was made to feel the seasons. To sense the cold and respond to it. But most of us live at one temperature now - indoors, wrapped, protected, and disconnected. We've forgotten what cold is for.

This is not about toughness. Cold isn't here to punish you. It's here to wake something up. To remind your cells how to generate warmth from within. To teach your mitochondria how to work, how to burn clean, efficient, and strong.

The Function

Cold exposure builds resilience. It strengthens the mitochondria. When you're cold, your body doesn't just shiver, it activates. It turns on fat-burning. It boosts blood flow. Improves oxygen use. Stabilises blood sugar. And clears inflammation.

When you pair it with morning light or natural elements like ocean water, you give your body a stronger signal, "This is morning. This is the season I'm in." Your nervous system calms. Your mood shifts. Your system learns to face the day with strength.

The Fracture

We stopped feeling cold. Heaters, hot showers, layers of clothes. We traded adaptability for comfort. Now our bodies overheat. Our immune systems overreact. Our mitochondria have weakened from lack of use.

We forgot that stress isn't always bad. The right kind of stress creates strength. Your body was made to move through cold, not to fear it.

The Return

Start gently. Let the cold in slowly. No force. Just consistency.

If You're New to Cold

- **Wash your face and neck |** With cold water after waking.
- **Step outside barefoot |** 1 - 2 minutes each morning. Let your skin feel the cool air.
- **Finish your morning shower with cold |** Start with 30 seconds, slowly build to 2 minutes.
- **Leave a window open |** Cool the body naturally while you move or stretch inside.
- **Let your body cool gently after activity |** Don't rush to layer up.

If You're Ready for More

- **Try cold ocean dips |** Saltwater helps ground your body. Rivers, lakes, or a simple cold bath at home work great too.
- **Submerge up to the neck |** Let the cold wrap around you.
- **Stay until the breath calms |** Then a little longer. Walk out if your breath becomes jagged.
- **Breathe slow into the cold |** Try 4 seconds in, 6 seconds out. This calms the nervous system and feeds your mitochondria with oxygen.
- **Pair with the sunrise |** Receive the light with skin still tingling from the cold.

- **Let your body rewarm naturally |** Move gently afterward, walking, stretching. Skip the hot shower straight away.

Tips

- **Wear a thermal swim cap or beanie |** They help to retain heat on those particularly cold mornings.
- **Wear booties and gloves in Winter |** If the water is especially cold, they help protect your hands and feet from deep chill.

***Important Note:** It's not about being extreme. Let breath lead, not ego. If you have a health condition or any doubts, check with a trusted professional first. If you're unwell, pause, and return when you're better.*

Signs of Restoration

You'll know the cold is working not by how hard it was, but by how you feel after. You step out clearer, sharper, more awake. Not just in body, but in mind.

Your breath deepens naturally. There's more energy, but less rush. You're not burning out by midday. Sleep becomes deeper at night, like your body trusts it can finally let go. Your hands and feet begin to warm themselves quicker, without needing help. And something shifts, cold no longer feels like an attack. It feels like an invitation.

Seasonal Shift

Spring | Lengthen exposure gently. Let the body stretch its resilience.
Summer | Use morning cold to sharpen energy. Let your body experience cool in contrast to heat.

Cold Strengthens the Cell

If your cell membranes, the insulation, become too loose or inflamed, they start to leak. This is called "membrane instability," and it underlies more conditions than we realise *(see pages 13 - 16 to refresh)*. This can happen for many reasons, but one not mentioned yet is if the body holds, or is exposed to, too much heat.

Cold helps to stabilise and seal the cell membranes by strengthening the fats that make up their structure. When those membranes hold strong, your circuit is steady. Inflammation settles. And peace can return.

Autumn | Build tolerance steadily as the water cools. Strengthen your internal fire before deep Winter.

Winter | This is where cold matters most. Short focused exposure followed by movement to gently rewarm.

Let cold wake what comfort put to sleep.

Build Strength

Load your system to build capacity.

Strength was never just about muscles. It was about stability. About having something inside you that doesn't shake when life gets heavy. Strength says, "I can hold this. I don't collapse here."

But most of us don't feel strong anymore. We feel drained. Brittle. We feel the weight of things more than we used to. And deep down, many of us have forgotten that strength isn't something we chase, it's something we return to. Your body was made to carry strength. Not bulk. Not image. But steady, resilient, mitochondrial strength.

The Function

When you use your muscles, especially under load, your mitochondria turn on. They burn. They multiply. Strength training isn't for size. It sharpens energy use. It makes your system more efficient and less fragile. It protects your bones, your brain, your nervous system.

And maybe most importantly, it rebuilds your trust in your body. Each rep says, "I'm not afraid of effort." Each step says, "I can hold more than I thought." Strength makes room for resilience to return.

The Fracture

We turned strength into appearance. We made it about abs and aesthetics instead of function. We chased 'burn' over balance. Overtrained. Under rested. Treated exercise like punishment for food instead of praise for life. And we forgot the kind of strength that builds from the inside out.

> ## Breath Stokes the Fire
>
> Your mitochondria don't run on light and food alone. They run on oxygen, delivered by your breath. If you hold your breath during cold exposure, during exercise, or if your breathing is shallow, rushed, or stuck - your mitochondria never fully turn on. Your body stays in low-power mode, conserving rather than burning.
>
> Breathe deep. Breathe wide. Not just to calm your nervous system, but to feed your fire during this phase. You don't need techniques here, just awareness. Let your breath rise through your ribs. Let your shoulders stay soft. Let your lungs stretch. Let the oxygen in. Because when you do, the mitochondria can burn.

Then we stopped moving. We sat all day. Let our posture collapse. Let our grip fade. We outsourced strength to automation, machines, and motors. But our bodies weren't made to be idle.

The Return

Start with permission. Not punishment. You don't need a gym to begin.

- **Lift something |** Water jugs, logs, your own body. Add resistance in small ways. It doesn't need to be complicated.
- **Do functional movements |** Squats, carries, pushes, pulls. Movements your ancestors would recognise.
- **Use your bodyweight |** Planks, lunges, bridges, push-ups. You can build strength without equipment.

- **Train your grip** | Hold, squeeze, carry. Grip strength is linked to longevity.
- **Go slow sometimes** | Slower reps build tension and control. Making muscles work harder and teaching your body steadiness.
- **Exhale through the effort** | Let your breath lead the movement. Inhale as you prepare, exhale as you lift.
- **Strength train 2 - 3x per week** | With recovery in between. A 10 - 20 minute session is enough. Consistency is key.
- **Don't fear rest** | Recovery is where strength roots. Without rest, training breaks you down instead of building you up.
- **Anchor it to rhythm** | Tie strength to light, to breath, to season. Let it weave in, not dominate.

Signs of Restoration

Your posture shifts. Your back holds upright without effort. You feel more solid in your steps. Your grip steadies. You don't fatigue as quickly. You carry things, groceries, children, stress, with less collapse. Even your thoughts feel stronger. You're remembering that you already carry strength.

Seasonal Shift

Spring | Begin with bodyweight. Walk hills. Do gentle strengthening after Winter's stillness.
Summer | Build intensity. Lift heavier. Let your energy meet the long light.
Autumn | Slow down the reps. Think stability, not volume.
Winter | Maintain. Use strength to keep the mitochondria burning. Short, intentional sessions.

You were designed to bear weight.

Optional Support | CoQ10

Coenzyme Q10 (CoQ10) is a compound your body makes naturally. It lives in the mitochondria. Its job is simple but vital. Help your cells turn food and oxygen into usable energy. Some people make less of it, especially as they get older, if they're under chronic stress or inflammation, or when taking cholesterol-lowering medication (like statins).

When CoQ10 levels are low, energy production slows. Fatigue lingers. Recovery takes longer.

You can support your body's levels through real food (like organ meats, oily fish, beef). But some people also explore supplements if food alone isn't enough. This can be especially relevant if you're on statins, or if you've done all the core mitochondrial supports and still feel flat.

If supplementing:

- **Look for ubiquinol (the active form) |** Not ubiquinone.
- **Take with fat |** Ideally in the morning.
- **Don't use it to push harder |** Use it to restore gently.
- **Doses of 100 - 200 mg are typical |** Enough to restore, not to overdrive. Once energy steadies and recovery feels strong, you may drop to a maintenance dose of 50 - 100 mg.

Restorative Light

Let healing light return to your cells.

Red light doesn't just shine, it enters. It moves past skin, past the surface. Down to the mitochondria where energy is made. You might've heard the term and thought it was a trend. But this isn't new. Your body has always known this light. The reds of firelight. The low sun at dawn and dusk. The warmth of light that doesn't stimulate, but restores. Red light therapy (RLT) is a way to bring that light back in.

The Function

Red and near-infrared light (typically 620 - 860 nm) absorbs into the mitochondria. When this light hits them, the mitochondria become more efficient. They burn cleaner. They heal faster.

It reduces inflammation. Supports muscle recovery. Improves skin texture and collagen. Strengthens circulation. Speeds wound healing. Balances hormones.

But it's not just physical. Red light therapy brings the body into a calm, ready state. It reminds the system, you're safe to repair now. Where blue light speeds things up, red light guides you back.

The Fracture

We used to live in rhythm with the sun, light in the morning, dark at night. Firelight to close the day. But we swapped it for LEDs, screens, and fluorescents. Bright white light all day. Blue glare all night. This overexposure told our cells to stay alert. Don't repair. Don't rest.

And then we got sick more often. Slept less. Healed slower. The kind of light our cells once trusted, disappeared. We didn't just lose natural darkness. We lost restorative light.

Sunlight vs Red Light Therapy Panels

Sunrise & Sunset | 1 - 5 mW/cm² | Red light is gentle in strength. It works to set your body clock, and calm your nervous system. The dose is small but powerful for rhythm.

Midday Sun | 30 - 50 mW/cm² | Red light is strong, matching the strength of a panel session but with the added benefits of natural charge and vitamin D.

RLT Panels | 50 - 150 mW/cm² | The concentrated red and infrared light delivers an efficient dose in just a few minutes, without UV. Ideal if you can't get sunlight daily, or for treating specific areas.

Bottom Line | Panels deliver a controlled dose of what the sun gives you. They're a tool, not a substitute. Sunrise and sunset tune your clock. Midday sun delivers raw power. Panels fill in the gaps when natural light isn't enough.

Making Sense of the Numbers

When people talk about red light therapy, you'll see two units:

mW/cm² (milliwatts per square centimetre) | Think of this as how strong the light is - the power hitting your skin at any moment. Like the speed of water coming out of a hose.

J/cm² (joules per square centimetre) | This is the total dose you've received - the energy that actually lands in your body. Like how much water fills the bucket after the hose has been running for a while.

The Return

- **Start with the real thing** | Step into morning, midday, and evening light first. Natural light is the original therapy. Use panels to fill the gaps - when weather, season, or work keep you indoors.
- **Use an RLT device in the morning or early evening** | When red light pairs well with sunrise and sunset, anchoring circadian rhythm. See "Choosing a Red Light Device" on page 226.
- **Breathe slowly** | RLT works best when your body is in rest mode. Inhale gently, then exhale a little longer. Calm breathing tells your body it's safe, and opens your cells to receive.
- **Shine it on the face, chest, joints or muscles** | Focus on areas that need recovery or repair. Red light helps reduce inflammation, restore tissue, and support adaptation after training.
- **Don't stare into the light** | Keep eyes closed or use tinted goggles.
- **More is not always better** | There's a sweet spot, and it changes depending on your body and device. Start small with just 1 - 2 minutes. Listen to your body before increasing.

Signs of Restoration

Your skin starts to carry a soft glow. Muscles recover faster, with less soreness after effort. Sleep comes easier and feels deeper. Inflammation settles. Hormones shift toward balance. And through it all, your energy begins to rise, not sharply, but steadily, like a low hum returning to your system.

Finding Your Red Light Dose

Times are approximate for a *100 mW/cm² device* - adjust shorter for stronger devices, and longer for weaker.

Dose	Time	Typical Use	Why It Helps
5 J/cm²	50 sec	Skin-level: acne, wound healing, hair growth, skin inflammation	Activates cells in the top skin layers, boosts collagen, calms irritation
20 J/cm²	3 min 20 sec	Shallow tissue: fascia, small muscles, nerves, circulation	Energises mitochondria, improves blood flow, and repair
40 J/cm²	6 min 40 sec	Deeper tissue: large muscles, joints, tendons, pain relief	Reaches further into tissue, supports recovery reduces inflammation,

Seasonal Shift

Spring | Use red light to support detox and cellular renewal. Regular short morning sessions work best.

Summer | Prioritise natural light over devices. The natural sunrise and midday sun is often enough at this time of year.

Autumn | Begin layering in red light therapy as outdoor exposure reduces. Combine it with relaxed abdominal breathing.

Winter | Use red light daily, mornings especially. It helps fill the gap when natural light is dim.

Let the light remind the body, you're allowed to heal now.

Phase 4 | Rhythm Checklist

This month is about sparking the fire inside the cell with cold, strength and restorative light. Start where you feel ready. Be gentle, take your time.

Cold

- ☐ Splash your face with cold water on waking.
- ☐ Stand outside with bare skin in the morning for 1 - 2 minutes.
- ☐ Finish showers cold. Start with 30 seconds, build to 2 minutes.
- ☐ Combine cold with your breath (inhale 4, exhale 6).
- ☐ Try a brief ocean dip or cold bath up to the neck. Stay until breath steadies, then 30 - 60 seconds longer.

Strength

- ☐ 2 - 3 short sessions per week (10 - 20 minutes). Rest between days.
- ☐ Focus on functional movements - squat, hinge, push, pull, carry, hang.
- ☐ Use bodyweight or simple weights (water jugs, dumbbells, kettlebells).
- ☐ Go slow on some reps - feel control through full range.
- ☐ Stop 1 - 2 reps before form breaks.
- ☐ Inhale to prepare, exhale on effort.

Restorative Light

- ☐ Prioritise natural light - use devices to fill the gap.
- ☐ Time sessions to the sunrise or sunset.
- ☐ Aim light at face, chest, joints, or areas that need repair.
- ☐ Pair with slow, steady breathing.

Phase 4 | A Day in Rhythm

Morning

At sunrise, place your water in the light, then step outside barefoot, stretch while the sun rises. When you return, drink mineral-rich, structured water. Sit to a hearty breakfast. Mix a glass of electrolytes and sip it through the morning. Make the bed, open the windows.

In the shower, end with a burst of cold. Let it wake your mitochondria, sharpening your body's strength. Warm again with a short session of bodyweight work. Squats, lunges, planks, push-ups, simple holds. Ten minutes is enough. Sometimes, red light follows, supporting recovery and easing old injuries.

Midday

Pause to meet the sun. You stay a little longer these days, grounding if you can. Loosen with a short stretch. Sit down to lunch. Nourishing, unprocessed food, eaten without rush. The meal steadies you. Keep sipping water through the day, mineral-rich and clean. On hotter days, an extra electrolyte drink keeps the body charged.

Evening

Eat an early, light dinner. Eaten mindfully. Drink a glass of electrolytes, then head out for a walk at sunset, barefoot if possible, watching the light fade.

Back home, dim the lights, quiet the sound, switch off the tech. Sometimes you use red light here too, helping the body ease into night. Settle with broth and reading in a favourite chair, in a space that feels restful. When sleep is near, the bedroom is cool and dark, with natural bedding that lets the body breathe. In bed, five minutes of gentle breath reset softens you into sleep.

A Life in Rhythm | David's Fire Returns

David is 53. Six months ago, his cholesterol had crept up high enough that his doctor prescribed a statin. The numbers came down, but David began to feel like something else was slipping. He was tired in a way he hadn't been before. His muscles cramped, his legs ached, and even gentle exercises left him drained. He said it felt as if age had suddenly caught up to him. But David's problem wasn't age - it was energy. His mitochondria, the tiny engines in his cells, weren't burning well.

He began with small steps. At morning and midday, he stepped outside to catch the light, letting it soak into his skin. He added simple strength work - squats, planks, slow lifts - that didn't exhaust him but reminded his muscles how to move. He started using CoQ10 alongside his medication. And a few times each week, he walked into the cold ocean, letting the shock and saltwater wake something deeper in him.

Four weeks in, the difference was clear. His legs no longer cramped so easily. He could exercise without crashing the next day. Fatigue still came, but it no longer flattened him. He felt a spark returning - a sense that his body wasn't done yet.

Phase 5
Fuel the Fire

Length: ~ 6 - 8 weeks

Pillars Restored: Fire, Fat

Food is not the enemy. It's how you rebuild your fire.

This phase restores trust with food.

Let your body remember what real fuel feels like.

A Note Before We Begin

Before you read this chapter, pause. Take a breath. This section may challenge what you've believed about food, health, even morality. You might have been taught that a plant-heavy diet is "clean" or that animal foods should be a "last resort." That's understandable. A lot of those ideas have shaped how we see healthy eating.

But this chapter isn't here to argue. It's here to offer something deeper. A return to how humans once ate, before processed food, before agricultural overload, before metabolic collapse. This isn't a diet trend. It's a restoration of fuel. You don't have to agree with every word. Just read slowly. Let your body be part of the conversation.

When To Go Slowly

This chapter is a companion, not a prescription. Shifts in carbs and fat can change blood markers and medication needs. If you're pregnant, have a medical condition, or take daily prescriptions, make changes slowly with your clinician's guidance. If a change leaves you dizzy, nauseous, or unusually tired - pause, simplify, and check in. See the appendix for troubleshooting if you get stuck.

Introduction

This phase will feel different. You might notice the tone shift. It's firmer. More direct. Less poetic. That's on purpose. You're not just shifting habits here, you're changing fuel systems. This is metabolic ground zero.

Most people today are stuck in sugar mode. Burning fast, crashing often, and chasing energy from meal to meal. This phase breaks that cycle. It teaches your body to burn fat as its primary fuel, and to finally run with steady energy and clear thinking.

But to get there, you'll need to cut through a lot of confusion, food myths, marketing lies, and habits that feel normal but aren't helping. That's why the tone is sharper.

This isn't about being perfect. But it is about being honest. Some things you've been eating are draining you. Some things you've avoided are exactly what your body needs. Most people have never been taught what real fuel actually is. Let yourself read it slowly. Let it challenge you. You were never made to run on fumes. You were designed to burn steady and clean.

Return to Ancestral Fuel

Fat is the fuel your mitochondria prefer. It burns slowly and efficiently. It produces less waste, less inflammation, and more usable energy per molecule than carbohydrates. It keeps you stable in your mood, your hunger, your focus. When your body is running on fat, you don't crash. You don't need to snack every two hours. You stop chasing energy, because energy stays.

But somewhere along the way, we forgot that. We shifted to sugar, carbohydrates, and processed food. We told the body to run on quick energy, but that kind of fuel burns fast and fades fast. It leaves you hungry, tired, and inflamed.

Here's the Truth

You might be surprised how little carbohydrate you need. Your body can make the small amount of glucose it needs from protein and from fat. Your liver was designed for this. It's called gluconeogenesis. You were made to run on fat, and the body can take care of the rest.

When you return to ancestral fuel (high fat, moderate protein, low carb), everything begins to shift. Energy steadies instead of spiking and crashing. Cravings soften, no longer pulling you off course. The mind clears, inflammation settles, and the body can finally turn back to repair.

In the pages ahead, you'll be walked through what this looks like. What to eat. What to expect. And how to shift without crashing. But for now, just know this, you were never broken. You were just running on the wrong fuel.

You don't need more willpower. You need food that burns clean.

Opening the Pantry Again

Before we go further, we need to talk about food. Not just categories. But types, sources, and the way they've changed. In this next part, we're going to look at what's actually in our homes and on our plates. We'll walk through the different kinds of animal foods, the ones that build and repair, and the ones that do more harm than good. We'll look at plants, which ones support the body, and which ones might be draining your energy without you realising. We'll talk about oils and fats. We'll even touch on drinks, packaging, and how the way we cook and store food affects your body.

This isn't about fear. It's about clarity. It's time to open the pantry again, to lay it all out. And to let your body relearn what it was actually made to eat.

Let the pantry open with truth.

Not All Meat is the Same

Not all meat is the same. And not all animals were created to nourish us in the same way. Some give clean, steady fuel that helps the body repair. Others are harder to digest, more inflammatory, or carry what they've been fed. Knowing the difference matters if you want food that truly supports you.

Red Meat

The cleanest fuel for the human body comes from ruminant animals, like lamb, beef, goat, and venison. These animals have a multi-stage digestive system that naturally filters their food and builds nutrient-dense fat and tissue. Their meat tends to be better tolerated, more mineral-rich, and deeply nourishing for mitochondrial health.

Pork

Pork, though common, is different. Pigs don't have this filtering system. They're single-stomached animals that absorb more from their environment, including toxins and inflammatory compounds. For those trying to stabilise energy, reduce inflammation, or restore gut health, pork can be problematic.

Chicken

Chicken is often seen as a safe, lean protein, but it doesn't stabilise the system the way red meat can. While it can be tolerated by many, especially when pasture-raised and cooked simply, it doesn't offer the same mineral density, fat profile, or mitochondrial support as ruminant animals.

Many commercial chickens are raised in crowded environments and fed grains, which can alter the fat quality and introduce inflammatory compounds into their meat. The result is a fuel that feels light to eat, but not always cleaner. If you include chicken, prioritise organic, pasture-raised, and bone-in cuts. Use it in moderation, not as a foundation. It's not harmful by nature, but it's not as deeply nourishing as red meat. Let your body tell you how it responds.

Dairy

Dairy was designed to feed the young. Some bodies tolerate butter or ghee well. Others may do well with raw or fermented versions. But milk proteins and sugars can often trigger inflammation or gut issues, especially if consumed daily or in processed forms. Consider avoiding most dairy to begin with. Although butter and ghee are usually safe and a great source of fat.

Eggs

Eggs are nutrient-dense but also one of the most common food sensitivities. The yolk is typically better tolerated than the white. If your system is still healing, it's best to avoid them initially and then reintroduce eggs slowly and watch closely for any symptoms.

Seafood

Small oily fish (sardines, mackerel, herring, wild salmon). These fish are high in omega-3s, selenium, and trace minerals without the toxin load of larger fish.

Avoid shellfish, bottom-feeders, and filter feeders (prawns, mussels, oysters). They help clean the ocean, but they carry what they clean. If your body needs healing, they may introduce too many toxins.

What About Plants?

For years, we've been told that more plants equals better health. That a colourful plate is a sure sign of vitality. But here's the part no one explains. Plants are *not* passive. They *don't* want to be eaten. Unlike animals, they can't run or hide, so they defend themselves chemically.

Many common plants contain compounds like oxalates, lectins, phytates, salicylates, and tannins. Natural molecules that can irritate the gut, bind minerals, trigger inflammation, or disrupt mitochondrial function. These effects might be subtle at first like bloating, fatigue, stiff joints, or brain fog. But over time, they can become chronic and deeply problematic for some.

This doesn't mean all plants are harmful to all people. But it does mean they aren't neutral. And for those whose energy systems are already compromised, certain plant foods may do more harm than good. You don't have to fear plants. But you do need to understand them.

Grains

Grains like wheat, oats, barley, and corn became staples during times of survival. They store well, feed many, and provide quick calories. But that doesn't mean they're the best source of fuel.

Most grains contain compounds that can irritate the gut lining, spike blood sugar, or feed inflammation - especially when eaten daily or in processed forms. They don't offer much usable fat, and they often leave people feeling hungry again soon after eating.

If you're trying to rebuild energy, restore gut health, or stabilise your mitochondria, grains are best left off the plate, at least during recovery.

Root Vegetables

Root vegetables like potatoes, sweet potatoes, beets, and carrots are often seen as wholesome. And for some people, they can be tolerated. But roots are storage organs, they're built to hold starch and resist decay. That means they often contain compounds that can be irritating for people with digestive issues, autoimmune conditions, or energy instability.

If your mitochondria are still recovering, starch can interrupt the shift to clean-burning fuel. Some roots may return later, but in this phase, they're not essential.

Other Vegetables

Not all vegetables are the same, but most were not designed to be eaten in large daily amounts. Leafy greens (like spinach), cruciferous vegetables (like broccoli, kale and cauliflower), and nightshades (like tomatoes and capsicum) all contain defence chemicals.

Some bind minerals. Some affect the thyroid. Some inflame the gut. This doesn't mean you have to avoid all vegetables forever. But if your system is inflamed, tired, or reactive, it's wise to reduce. If they're interfering more than helping, it's okay to pause them while you heal.

A Note on Safer Plants

Your body isn't wrong if it reacts to plants. It may simply be responding to chemicals it was never designed to carry in excess. With time and repair, some people can return to carefully chosen plants in small amounts.

There's a section later in the book on how to reintroduce safely, if or when you're ready. For now, if you're in a healing phase, it's okay to pause most plant foods.

The following are generally better tolerated if introduced slowly, cooked well, and timed correctly:

- **Low-Toxin Veg |** Carrots, swede, turnip, zucchini, pumpkin
- **Low-Toxin Fruit |** Blueberries, pear, apple
- **Cold-Pressed Oils (occasionally) |** Olive oil, coconut oil
- **Herbs |** Rosemary, thyme, oregano

Be cautious with nuts, seeds, grains, legumes, leafy greens and nightshades. If it fogs, bloats, or scatters you, it's not the time.

Fruit

Fruit is beautiful, but it's seasonal. It was never meant to be available year-round or used to replace fat. Modern fruit is much higher in sugar than its wild ancestors and more concentrated than the body expects.

Fruit can be supportive for some, especially in warm seasons or after adaptation. But if you're trying to regulate energy, break food dependency, or lower inflammation, it's best to keep fruit minimal or paused for now.

Legumes

Beans, lentils, and peas are often promoted as health foods. But they contain lectins and other compounds that can irritate the gut, trigger bloating, and disrupt mineral absorption. They're also quite high in carbohydrates and require careful preparation to make them digestible through soaking, sprouting, and fermenting.

In this phase, while the body is recalibrating, legumes usually create more noise than clarity.

Nuts and Seeds

Nuts and seeds contain the beginning of life. Inside them is a plant, a tree, a forest. So they protect what they carry. They store antinutrients, enzyme inhibitors, and oils that oxidise quickly. Some people tolerate small amounts of well-prepared nuts or seeds, but many find they trigger bloating, skin issues, or cravings.

The Bottom Line

This isn't about fear. It's about clarity. Plants are complex. Some heal. Some harm. Some do both, depending on the body, the dose, and the timing.

You don't have to make a lifelong decision today. But while you're rebuilding your health, simplify. Focus on the foods that fuel you. Test gently. Add back slowly. Let your body lead through peace, not cravings.

Not all food is foundational. Some is optional. Some is occasional. But the core must be clean, steady, and clear. Let your body decide what stays.

Not all plants are fuel. Let your body show you which add peace.

Plant Compounds and Common Reactions

Not everyone reacts to these. But if your system is tired, inflamed, or healing, these compounds can make matters worse. This isn't about fear. It's about noticing.

	Where It's Found	Common Reactions
FODMAPs	Garlic, onion, apples, wheat, legumes	Gas, bloating, cramping, diarrhoea, constipation
Histamines & Histamine Liberators	Aged & fermented foods, spinach, avocado, strawberries, citrus	Headaches, migraines, skin rashes, itchy eyes, insomnia, anxiety-like symptoms
Lectins	Legumes, grains, nightshades, tomatoes, capsicum, eggplant	Bloating, joint pain, fatigue, immune reactivity
Oxalates	Spinach, beetroot, sweet potato, cacao, chia, soy, nuts, seeds, gluten-free flours, plant-based milks	Sharp joint or nerve pain, fibromyalgia-like pain, vulvodynia, bladder irritation, kidney stones, mineral loss
Phytates	Grains, nuts, seeds, legumes	Poor mineral absorption, fatigue, brittle nails, thin hair
Salicylates	Berries, herbs, honey, spices, many fruits	Headaches, skin rashes, hives, allergy-like symptoms, anxiety, hyperactivity
Tannins	Tea, red wine, legumes, nuts, some berries	Nausea, gut irritation, reduced iron absorption, tension headaches

Let's Talk About Fats and Oils

Not all fats are the same. Some stabilise your energy, support hormones, and help your body burn clean. Others disrupt your cells, confuse your digestion, and leave behind chaos your body has to mop up. The kind of fat you eat matters, especially if you're rebuilding from the inside out.

The Cleanest Fats for Fuel

The most supportive fats come from animals that graze, like lamb, beef, goat, and venison. They are **saturated fats:**

- **Beef Tallow |** Rendered beef fat.
- **Suet |** Hard raw beef fat near the kidneys.
- **Lamb Tallow |** Rendered lamb fat.
- **Lamb Fat |** Hard raw lamb fat.
- **Goat Fat |** Hard raw goat fat.

These fats are highly saturated, stable when heated, and deeply nourishing. They burn clean, giving you steady energy without adding inflammation or stress. They're also rich in fat-soluble vitamins and help strengthen cell membranes, making them less likely to leak or misfire. This is the kind of fat your mitochondria understand. Especially during healing, these are your best fuels.

Fats That May Be Tolerated

The following fats may work depending on your body and how much inflammation you're carrying. But they are not core fuels, use them carefully. Let your body speak.

> ## Fat Stores Light
>
> Sunlight doesn't just warm the skin. It enters nature. Plants capture light and seal it into molecules, into sugars, starches, and fats. Animals eat those plants. The light is stored again. And when you eat well-sourced fats, you're taking in light that has been stabilised and preserved ready for release.
>
> When you burn fat, that stored light is released. It becomes warmth. Motion. Charge. Repair. And some of that energy radiates back out.
>
> This gentle glow is what scientists call biophoton emission. Tiny flashes of light your cells release as they work. You were made to carry light. And to shine.

- **Duck fat |** Softer and richer than beef fat. Some thrive on it, others don't digest it well.
- **Butter and ghee |** Nutrient-dense, but dairy-based. Ghee is often well tolerated.
- **Pork fat or lard |** Can be more inflammatory than people realise. Best avoided if you're still healing.
- **Olive oil |** Raw, cold-pressed, un-heated, and only in small amounts.
- **Coconut oil |** Antimicrobial. May help during detox phases.
- **Avocado oil |** Can oxidise easily. If used, keep it cold and unheated.

The Ones to Remove

These fats, **polyunsaturated fats (PUFAs)**, don't belong in your kitchen or in your body: canola oil, soybean oil, sunflower oil, corn oil, grapeseed oil, rice bran oil, and vegetable oil blends.

They are liquid at room temperature, quick to break down, and unstable when heated. That fragility disrupts membranes, throws off hormonal signals, and creates byproducts that stress your cells. Even in small amounts, they cause chaos and promote inflammation.

The Bottom Line

Choose fats that are stable, not fragile. Look for what's solid at room temperature, not what's bottled in factories. These steady, ancestral fuels burn clean, support repair, and keep your energy even. Fragile, factory-made oils break apart and leave your body with more inflammation to clear.

Choose what burns clean and your body will remember how to steady.

Cholesterol | Nothing to Fear

You were never meant to fear cholesterol. Your body makes it, every single day. Not because something is wrong, but because something is right. Cholesterol is not a threat. It's a builder. A healer. A responder. It rises when the body is repairing, protecting, or restructuring.

What Cholesterol Actually Does:

- **Builds hormones |** Estrogen, progesterone, testosterone, cortisol.
- **Supports your brain |** 25% of your body's cholesterol is in your brain, where it helps with memory, learning and thinking.
- **Creates vitamin D |** Sunlight + Cholesterol = Vitamin D
- **Repairs tissue |** Acts like scaffolding in healing.
- **Forms bile |** Needed to break down and absorb fat.

... Continued

Why the Fear Started

Years ago, researchers blamed cholesterol for clogging arteries and causing heart attacks. But they were looking in the wrong place. Cholesterol was present, but not the cause. It was like blaming firefighters for the fire, just because they're always on the scene.

What Actually Causes Damage in the Arteries

- **Inflammation** | From processed food, PUFAs, sugar, stress.
- **Oxidised cholesterol** | If it's been damaged by toxins or excess sugar.
- **Calcium accumulation** | Due to low magnesium or vitamin K2.

What to Check Instead of Just "Total Cholesterol"

Total cholesterol doesn't tell you much. What matters more:

- **CRP (C-reactive protein)** | Low means low inflammation
- **LDL particle size** | Large/fluffy = safe. Small/dense = more risky
- **Fasting insulin and blood sugar** | Markers of metabolic health
- **Coronary Artery Calcium Score** | A zero score = no calcification

Final Note:

Cholesterol is not your enemy. If your levels rise after switching to real food, but the tests above are normal, don't panic. For many, that shift simply reflects repair - your body finally has the raw materials to rebuild membranes, hormones, and bile. Let peace return. Eat without fear. Your body knows what it's doing.

What You Drink Matters

We often think of fuel as food. But what you drink shapes your body just as much, sometimes more. Fluids decide whether your cells are hydrated and charged or scattered and dry.

Most people today aren't drinking enough water. Or worse, they're filling their bodies with sweetened, flavoured, or chemical-laden drinks. Your cells run on electrical charge, and water is what carries that charge. Without clean water, your body is running on static.

Water | Your Foundation

Still, mineral-rich water is the base. It's not just about drinking enough, it's about drinking the right kind. Your water should be:

- **Filtered** | To remove toxins and heavy metals.
- **Mineralised** | To replace what's stripped out.
- **Charged** | By light and movement.
- **Stored safely** | Avoid plastics or anything with a chemical taste.

Avoid flavoured waters, artificial sweeteners, or anything that doesn't leave you feeling hydrated.

What About Sparkling Water?

Some do well with natural sparkling water, especially mineral-rich ones. But if it bloats you or leaves your stomach unsettled, stick with still water. The simplest is usually the best.

Herbal Tea | Sometimes Supportive

Herbal teas can help, but not all of them. Some may soothe (like chamomile, peppermint, rooibos, or ginger), while others can overstimulate or interfere with your body's natural rhythms. Spicy detox blends or medicinal mixes are often too harsh if your system is already inflamed. Use herbal tea with intention, not out of habit.

Coffee and Caffeine

Coffee isn't bad, but it's often misused. It forces tired systems to push harder when they should be resting. It can spike cortisol, trigger cravings, and stop your energy from stabilising. If you're healing, it's wise to reduce or pause caffeine until your energy is steady. If you do drink it, keep it to one cup a day, in the morning, with food, not on an empty stomach.

Energy drinks, pre-workouts, or caffeine pills. Never. They leave the body more drained than before.

Alcohol

Alcohol scatters your rhythm and dulls your clarity. It weakens boundaries, disrupts sleep, and interferes with cellular repair. If you want your energy back, step away from alcohol completely while you heal. Later, a glass on special occasions might be tolerated, but it should never be a tool for numbing or coping.

Dairy-Based Drinks

Some adults do fine with small amounts, especially raw or fermented forms like kefir. But many experience bloating, inflammation, sinus congestion or skin flares. If you're using milk, milk-based smoothies, or flavoured milks, be careful. They're not foundational.

Milk Alternatives

Most plant milks aren't the clean alternative they claim to be. Almond milk, oat milk, soy milk, they're often loaded with gums, oxalates, phytates, seed oils, sugars, and additives that strain digestion and disrupt your gut. If you want an alternative, choose unsweetened coconut milk with minimal ingredients.

Juices and Smoothies

Juices, even cold-pressed ones, are just sugar water without the fibre. They spike your blood glucose, fuel cravings, and overwhelm your system.

Smoothies often mix too many things together, powders, sweeteners, and frozen fruit, which don't digest cleanly.

Your body was built to chew, not sip meals. Whole food, eaten slowly, is better recognised by your cells.

Fizzy Drinks, Cordials, and Soft Drinks

These drinks are a trap. Even the 'diet' versions scatter your energy, confuse your gut, and leave your body dehydrated. They interfere with energy regulation and feed inflammation. If you want to rebuild your system, remove them entirely.

Powdered Drinks and Supplements

Protein shakes, boosters, and 'health powders' are concentrated and often filled with additives. Some have a place during recovery, but most are overused, leaving people dependent on processed drinks instead of real food. If your energy is unstable, pause all powders until your health is steady.

The Bottom Line

Fluids aren't just hydration, they're signals. Some calm and carry life. Some stir chaos and block your body's ability to recharge. Choose clean water as your foundation. Let every other drink earn its place.

When the List Feels Like Too Much

You might feel it as you read through this phase, the tightening in your chest, the questions rising: *"Wait, I can't eat that? What's left?"*

That reaction is completely normal. But here's the truth. You're not being punished. You're being cleared. You've lived in a system that fed you confusion. It taught you to eat constantly, chase nutrients, balance charts, and live on snacks, supplements, and willpower.

This isn't that. This isn't a diet. It's a return. The food list might look short, but what it gives back is enormous. Clarity. Stillness. Steady energy. A body that stops shouting and starts listening.

You're not being restricted. You're being recalibrated. Not forever. Just long enough to remember what real fuel feels like.

How to Cook, Store, and Prepare Food

Food isn't just fuel. It's memory. It's energy. It's timing. How food is cooked, stored, or prepared, changes the way your body receives it. And most people don't realise, it's not just what's on the plate, but how it got there. It's about remembering what food was meant to be. Alive, clean, and nourishing.

Freshness First

The closer food is to its natural state, in time, texture, and form, the more support it gives. Fresh meat, fresh fat, and recently picked produce carry a kind of life your body recognises. But when food is frozen for months, stored too long, or packaged far from its source, that charge begins to dull.

Yes, freezing has its place. It helps reduce waste. But it slows the rhythm. Frozen food is paused food. If you can, keep your food rotation short. Buy what you'll eat soon. Let your meals echo the season you're in, not one from long ago.

How You Cook It Matters

Cooking isn't the problem. In fact, it can help make food safer, easier to digest, and even more supportive. But how you cook matters.

- **Cook with care |** Not rushed, not distracted.
- **Don't burn |** Don't boil hard or reheat constantly.
- **Be Gentle |** Use slow roasting, gentle simmering, or light searing.
- **Let meat rest |** Let flavours settle. Let it breathe.

Food that's been cooked too hard or too long loses its shape, not just physically, but energetically. You want food that's still recognisable in your body. Still intact.

Fermented Foods | Helpful or Harmful?

Fermentation has been praised for gut health, and sometimes rightly so. But not all fermented foods are helpful. And not all bodies tolerate them.

Some fermentation helps (when done well) by breaking down fibre and adding beneficial bacteria. Ferments that may be tolerated by some include fresh coconut yoghurt, lightly fermented vegetables, and water kefir. On the other hand, stronger or longer ferments - or those your body doesn't tolerate - can cause bloating or trigger immune reactions. Be especially cautious with kombucha, kimchi, sauerkraut, and fermented dairy or soy products.

Fermented foods aren't required. Some may support the body during specific phases. Use discernment, not trend. If they stir symptoms or leave your system inflamed or foggy, step away.

Preserved Meats

Preserved meats like jerky or cured cuts can be helpful at certain times like travel. But most supermarket versions are filled with sugar, seed oils, additives, and nitrates. Look for preserved meats that are:

- Sugar-free.
- Free from seed oils and preservatives.
- Made with simple ingredients. Meat, salt, herbs.
- Air-dried or gently smoked. Not chemically processed.

Storage and Shelf Life

There's wisdom in being prepared, but not in panic. Long-term food storage is only helpful if it's still alive and holds energy. When food is kept too long, it begins to lose its memory. And when we eat it, we feel that disconnection.

If it never spoils, if you can't smell its origin, it's likely lost its place. Your senses will know. Let them guide you. If you have to convince yourself it's healthy, it probably isn't.

The Bottom Line

Eat food that's recent, real, and respected. Cook it gently. Store it calmly. Eat it while its memory is still fresh. What you eat should match your body's rhythm, and your body's season.

It's not just what you eat, it's how it's handled.

Histamine | The Reason You May Still Feel Off

You're eating clean. Cooking from scratch. Avoiding the obvious triggers. But something still isn't right. Maybe you feel foggy after meals. Tired but can't sleep. Maybe your heart races, your skin itches, your gut won't settle, or your mood swings for no clear reason. You've cut the sugar, but your body still feels like it's always on edge. This might be histamine.

Histamine is a natural chemical your body makes. It's part of your immune system, a messenger. But if your system is already overloaded or inflamed,

... Continued

histamine can build up faster than your body can clear it. And when that happens, even healthy foods can tip things over the edge.

What Increases Histamine Load?

- Meals and broth cooked too long (over 2 hours).
- Leftovers (histamine builds up even when frigerated).
- Pre-packaged mince (the high surface area speeds up breakdown).
- Aged, smoked, canned, and processed meats.
- Cheeses and fermented foods. Sauerkraut, kombucha, vinegar.
- Avocado, spinach, tomatoes, and eggplant.
- Chocolate, black tea, green tea, and alcohol.

If your body is inflamed or reactive, these foods may add noise your system can't handle right now. Start by eating fresh, limiting aged or fermented items, and keeping meals simple. Often, just removing the build-up is enough for things to settle.

(See "What's Going on with Histamine and Allergies?" on page 16)

Choosing Your Starting Point

You've made it through the hardest part, letting go of old food rules. Now, it's time to rebuild. There isn't one single way to do this. Your body, your history, and your needs are unique. What follows are three paths. Each a different way of returning to fuel that's steady, simple, and clean. None are rules to lock into forever. They're starting points. Doorways. Some people need the deepest reset, some find balance with simplicity, and others do best with a little flexibility. Read them slowly, notice which one feels like relief, and begin there. You can always shift later. And remember, this isn't forever, foods can be added back. But while you are healing, simplicity is often best.

Option 1 | Animal-Based | Supportive + Flexible

This option is for those who feel better with a little more flexibility. It's rooted in animal foods, but makes space for small amounts of low-toxin plants. Think of it as supportive rather than strict. Ancestral in feel, modern in practice. It gives your body clear, steady fuel while allowing for a bit of variety. Done well, it still avoids the pitfalls of most modern diets while keeping things sustainable long term.

Examples of Meals

- Lamb ribs with avocado and sea salt.
- Grilled salmon with ghee and cucumber slices.
- Slow-cooked beef with roasted pumpkin.
- Chicken thighs with avocado and lettuce.
- Eggs scrambled in butter, with a few fermented carrots.

- Steak with a small side of grilled zucchini.
- Bunless beef burgers with avocado, lettuce and homemade mayo.

Option 2 | Standard Carnivore | Clean Simplicity

This is where many people find their groove. It keeps food simple: meat, fish, eggs, butter, animal fats. No plants, but plenty of variety within the animal kingdom. For many, this is what's needed to clear brain fog, reduce inflammation, and build steady energy. It's clean, grounding, and straightforward. Meals are easy to prepare and deeply satisfying. You'll find yourself eating two or three times a day without cravings, without the rollercoaster.

Examples of Meals

- Lamb cutlets with sea salt and ghee.
- Roasted chicken thighs cooked in tallow, with crispy skin, a side of butter and egg yolks.
- Wild salmon grilled in ghee, served with egg yolks.
- Slow cooked beef ribs with drippings.
- Scrambled eggs with extra yolks cooked in butter.
- Skin-on chicken thighs poached in salted water and served in their own broth. Soothing when you're unwell or need something light.

Option 3 | Lion Diet | Deep Healing

If you're dealing with autoimmune issues, chronic pain, or deep fatigue, sometimes you need to go further. The Lion Diet is the simplest reset. No plants, no dairy, no eggs. Just fresh ruminant meat, salt, and water. Nothing else. It sounds extreme, but for some, it's the doorway back to health. You won't stay here forever, but if your system is crashing, this can give it space to repair.

Keeping it Low-Histamine

The Lion Diet is also best kept low histamine, or it may backfire. The freshness of your meat matters. Beef is often hung for weeks, while lamb is usually much fresher. Find out when your butcher breaks down the meat. Order a week's worth, portion it up, and freeze it the same day. Only take out what you need. You can even cook straight from frozen. An air fryer or pressure cooker is excellent for this. Quick cooking (less than 60 minutes) keeps histamine low and your system calm.

Examples of Meals

- Pressure-cooked lamb shoulder with salt.
- Pan-fried lamb cutlets in tallow.
- Lamb belly strips crisped in the air fryer.
- Pan-fried steak with a side of roasted bone marrow. (Unaged beef)
- BBQ bone-in lamb chops, salted.
- Lamb mince patties cooked in the air fryer. (Use freshly ground mince from a butcher, not pre-packed.)

If You're Staying Lion for a While

If this way of eating feels right for you - you can stay here. Just remember that the longer you eat this way, the more important it becomes to support your vitamin and mineral levels. You can do this by adding a broad trace mineral supplement and including liver (or a liver supplement). Notice how you feel. If energy dips, it's not a setback, it's your body asking for a little extra support. If you're unsure, talk with a trusted practitioner.

Choose the path that steadies you.

Not Everyone Loves Liver

Organs are some of the most nutrient-dense foods on Earth. The original "superfoods". Liver, especially, is loaded with B12, folate, zinc, copper, vitamin K, CoQ10 and more. They support mitochondrial repair, nervous system function, and hormone balance. Eating "nose to tail" - not just muscle meat, but organs, fat, connective tissue, and bone - brings balance. It's how animals were meant to nourish us, providing the full spectrum of minerals and vitamins in the right ratios.

But not everyone can tolerate liver or wants to eat it every week. That's where clean, freeze-dried organ supplements can help.

Tips if supplementing

- **Choose grass-fed, freeze-dried capsules |** With no fillers. You want the organ and nothing else.
- **Take with fat for absorption |** Organs are rich in fat-soluble vitamins. Pairing them with fat helps your body absorb what's inside.
- **Dose |** Around 4 - 6 capsules per day is common. Always start lower if you're sensitive and build up gradually.
- **Include other organs too |** Adding in heart, kidney, or spleen broadens the nutrient profile and supports balance.

Build Meals That Burn Clean

What follows is a way to build meals that don't leave you foggy, inflamed, or flat. You're not eating to control your body anymore. You're eating to charge it. To feed your mitochondria.

The Ratio That Works

You don't need to track forever, but knowing the right ballpark helps when you're learning. A clean-burning, fat-fuelled meal looks like:

- 70 - 85% of calories from fat
- 15 - 25% of calories from protein
- 0 - 5% of calories from carbohydrates

That means your plate might not look 'balanced' the way you're used to. It will look denser. Simpler. And that's exactly right. That doesn't mean piling butter on top of everything, it means choosing naturally fatty cuts so the fat is built into the meal.

A Simple Guide to Portions

While you're learning, it can help to track for a short time. A free app, like Cronometer, makes it simple to check your fat, protein and carbohydrate intake until you get a feel for it. Once you know what your meals look like, you won't need the app, your body will guide you.

Protein | Protein is essential. Aim for around 1.0 - 1.5 grams per kilo of your ideal body weight (e.g. 80 - 120g/day for an 80kg person. Around 320 - 480 calories). This is enough to repair, recover and keep muscle.

Fat | Build the rest of your meal from fat. A good starting point is 2 - 3 times your protein intake in grams (e.g. 160 - 240g/day for someone eating 80g of protein. Around 1,440 - 2160 calories). This will feel like a lot to start, but over time, your body will adapt, and what first felt heavy will become steady and light.

Carbohydrate | If you're including some plants in your diet, aim to stay under 30 grams of carbohydrates per day (around 120 calories). This helps keep your body in fat-burning mode. With time, some people do well with a little more (up to about 100 grams), and still feel calm and balanced.

How to Adjust

Note that these numbers are just a starting point. Let appetite, energy, and recovery, be your guide. Here are a few simple signals to use.

- Constipated, hungry, cold, anxious, or low on energy → *add more fat.*
- Diarrhoea, heavy, nauseous or sluggish after meals → *reduce fat.*
- Feel weak, not recovering, or lose muscle → *add more protein.*
- Blood sugar feels jumpy or cravings spike → *reduce protein.*
- Flat during or after exercise → *add a little carbohydrate.*
- Cravings return or energy dips after adding carbs → *reduce carbs.*

Stop Overfeeding Protein

Most people trying to eat 'healthier' fall into the same trap. They eat too much protein, not enough fat, and feel worse than before. Here's why:

- **Too much protein = too much sugar |** Your liver converts the extra protein into glucose. This raises blood sugar and insulin, making you feel tired, inflamed, and craving more food.

- **Protein is not your main fuel** | It's for structure, not for energy.
- **It can strain digestion and your system** | Especially if your body is already depleted.

You're not meant to run on protein. You're meant to build with it. That's a very different job.

How to Increase Fat Without Feeling Sick

When your body has run on carbohydrates for years, switching fuels takes time. You may even feel foggy or flat at first. Here's how to gently increase fat so your digestion and system keep up:

- **Go slowly** | Add fat steadily over 2 - 4 weeks, not overnight.
- **Cook meat in tallow, suet, or ghee** | To gently layer fat in.
- **Start with less fatty cuts** | Beef rump, chicken thighs, salmon.
- **Chew slowly, eat calmly** | Fat digests best when you're relaxed.
- **Eat warm, cooked food** | This eases the digestive load.
- **Salt generously to taste** | Sodium and chloride from salt help support bile flow and stomach acid, both are key for digesting fat.
- **Broth primes digestion** | Drink a small amount before your meal.
- **Digestive Support** | If fat feels heavy or digestion is slow, a few simple additions may help. Try apple cider vinegar, a digestive enzyme with lipase, or ox bile/bile salts with meals. They can support you during the transition - especially if you've had your gallbladder removed.

Remember. There's no rush. Don't push through nausea or force it. If it feels wrong, pause, reassess, and come back to basics - salt, hydration, light, sleep.

Protein builds the frame. Fat lights the fire.

Choosing Foods by Fat Content

Most meats, even fatty ones, don't reach 70 - 85% fat by calories. These numbers are approximate and based on *cooked* values. Build meals around cuts that naturally carry fat, and add more when they don't

	Fat Percentage in Calories	Notes
Lamb Flap	75 - 80%	Ideal. Fat-dominant. Rich and sustaining.
Egg Yolk	75 - 80%	Great for boosting meals that are lower in fat.
High Fat Beef Mince (70/30)	70 - 75%	Good staple food option. Available from your local butcher.
Beef Brisket	65 - 70%	Rich in fat. But pour the drippings back over.
Lamb Shoulder	65 - 70%	Holds fat well. Good daily option. But still add extra - butter, tallow.
Whole Egg	60 - 65%	Leaner than it seems. Add extra yolks or fat.
Regular Beef Mince (80/20)	55 - 60%	Will likely need added fat. Fat can often cook out, pour it back on.
Salmon (skin-on)	55 - 60%	Protein heavy. Works best with added fat.
Ribeye / Scotch Steak	50 - 55%	Fatty cut but not enough alone. Pair with marrow or ghee.
Chicken Thigh (skin-on)	45 - 50%	Decent, but still protein heavy. Can be good for a lighter meal.

The Meal is More than What's on the Plate

You've just learned what to eat. But how you eat still matters just as much. Because food isn't only fuel, it's a signal. Every bite tells your body something. A rushed meal, eaten standing at the counter or scrolling on your phone, lands hard, unsettled. A meal eaten calmly, with your nervous system softened, lands completely differently.

Digestion doesn't begin in your stomach. It begins in your breath, your posture, your state of mind. If you come to the table tense and scattered, your gut tightens too. If you come open and steady, your body receives.

Try this next time you eat:

- Sit down. Not rushing, not standing.
- Turn off the screen. Let your attention be here.
- Place both feet on the ground. Feel held.
- Take a few slow breaths before beginning. Be thankful.
- Let your body land before the food does.

When you eat in rhythm, your gut softens. Your brain quiets. Your cells recognise the food as safe and nourishing. And your mitochondria, those tiny engines, can receive what you're feeding them.

It's about remembering that meals aren't just about nutrients, but about rhythm, calm, and connection.

The Reintroduction Roadmap

You've come this far. You've cleared the noise. Your body is finally humming again. Now comes the most delicate part. Deciding what, if anything, to bring back in.

Do You Even Need To?

You don't have to reintroduce anything. The meal is no longer about variety, it's about vitality. And you're allowed to protect that. Some people feel best staying on a simple animal-based, high-fat diet for life. That is allowed. That is enough.

But, if you want to, if your body feels strong, stable, and truly ready, you may try other foods. Not to 'go back to normal,' but to find a new normal that still holds your health.

How Do You Know You're Ready?

It's about stability. You're looking for steady energy and health. If even one of these is still shaky, wait. Rushing will blur the results.

- o Your digestion is calm and regular.
- o Your sleep is deep and steady.
- o You wake with energy and clarity.
- o Your cravings are gone.
- o Inflammation, pain, or fatigue have resolved.
- o You've had at least 4 - 6 solid weeks of baseline eating (longer for chronic issues).

How to Reintroduce

If you choose to reintroduce, keep it gentle. The slower you go, the clearer the signal will be.

- One food at a time.
- Small portion (e.g. 1 - 2 bites for the first meal).
- Eat a small amount once a day for 3 days, observing calmly.
- No other changes during this window. No new supplements, no new foods.
- If there are no symptoms, you can trial a slightly larger portion.
- If any symptoms arise - stop! Don't justify. Stop.
- Keep it slow. This is not a race.

Keep a Simple Food Diary and Symptom Log

This is optional, but powerful. Jot down:

- What you reintroduced.
- How you prepared it.
- How you felt over the next 3 - 5 days.

Watch For These Signs

If any of these appear, that food may not be safe yet. Listen gently. Symptoms can be immediate or delayed up to 3 - 5 days.

- Headaches, brain fog, fatigue
- Cravings & mood changes (irritability, sadness, anxiety)
- Sinus congestion
- Bloating, reflux, loose stools
- Joint pain, stiffness
- Skin issues, itching, flushing

Which Foods Are Least Reactive?

These are common safe optional reintroductions for many people. But don't treat this as a fixed list. Any food can be tested gently.

Animal Foods

- Butter and ghee
- Egg yolks
- Whole eggs
- A2 dairy (A2 cow's milk, goat or sheep milk, fresh goat or sheep cheese, sheep yoghurt)

Vegetables

- Lettuce, cucumber, zucchini, pumpkin
- Root vegetables: carrot, swede, turnip

Fruits

- Apple, pear, blueberries
- Avocado and avocado oil
- Olives and olive oil
- Coconut, coconut cream and coconut oil

Herbs

- Rosemary, thyme, oregano

Sweetener

- Honey. Small amounts only.

What If It Goes Badly?

That's not failure. That's information. Pull back. Return to baseline. Wait a few weeks. Try again later if you want to. Each step is information, not defeat.

You don't owe anyone a 'normal' plate.
You owe your body peace. Let that be the measure now.

Phase 5 | Rhythm Checklist

This phase rebuilds calm energy with clean fat, and simple meals. Most need 6 - 8 weeks to steady, though some may need longer - follow your own pace.

Pantry Reset

- ☐ Remove seed oils - canola, soybean, sunflower, corn, rice bran, grapeseed, vegetable blends, margarine. Read labels carefully. They often hide in dressings, sauces, and snacks.
- ☐ Clear ultra-processed foods, protein powders, flavoured drinks, cordials, soft drinks, and alcohol.
- ☐ Keep simple fats on hand - tallow, suet, ghee, butter.
- ☐ Stock fresh ruminant cuts that naturally carry fat - lamb, ribs, beef brisket, high fat mince. Buy fresh and freeze portions the same day.
- ☐ Keep plants minimal or paused. If including any, choose low-toxin options in small portions - zucchini, pumpkin, carrot, swede, turnip, cucumber, lettuce, apples, pears, blueberries.
- ☐ Avoid grains, legumes, nuts, seeds, and most leafy greens.

Building Meals

- ☐ Choose your starting point - animal based, carnivore or lion diet.
- ☐ Aim for roughly 70 - 85% of calories from fat, 15 - 25% from protein, 0 - 5% from carbs. Begin with an app like Cronometer to help initially.
- ☐ Choose a high fat animal food as the base for your meal.
- ☐ If including plants, keep carbs under ~ 30 grams a day.
- ☐ Use salt to taste and hydrate with mineralised water.

Phase 5 | A Day in Rhythm

Morning

At sunrise, carry your water outside to charge in the light. Barefoot, stretch on the grass while you watch the sunrise. When you return, drink a glass of mineral-rich, structured water.

Sit down to a hearty breakfast. High-fat, animal-based food, cooked with care. Afterwards, take electrolytes to steady and charge your body.

If there's space in the morning, you head to the ocean. A cold dip to teach your body to endure and burn from within. When time is shorter, you finish your shower with a burst of cold. Then, a short session of bodyweight strength. Ten minutes is enough to warm and energise you. Red light often follows, supporting energy and recovery.

Midday

You pause to meet the sun. First your front, then your back, grounding if you can. You let your body loosen with a short stretch. Sit to a full but simple lunch. Food is high-fat and nourishing. It steadies you. No need for snacks.

Evening

In the evening you might have a light dinner. Other nights, your body is still satisfied, so dinner is small, or even skipped altogether. After eating, you take a glass of electrolytes, and then walk at sunset, barefoot, watching the light fade.

You dim the lights, switch off the tech and relax with warm broth and reading. When you're ready for sleep, the bedroom is dark, cool, and layered with natural bedding. In bed, five minutes of relaxed breathing softens you into sleep.

> ### A Life in Rhythm | Sarah's Turning Point
>
> Sarah is 24 and suffers from swollen, painful joints. Her GP suspected early arthritis, possibly autoimmune, and was weighing up stronger medication. Sarah wasn't against it, but she was worried - her family history was full of autoimmune disease, and she wanted to know if there was anything else she could do alongside.
>
> Her story didn't stop at her joints. She also lived with bloating, eczema, and constant food reactions. Meals left her fatigued and foggy, yet she'd been told her diet had nothing to do with her joint pain. Deep down she wasn't convinced.
>
> After trying many approaches without much change, Sarah decided to try an animal-based diet - simple, low-histamine foods built around meat and fat. It wasn't easy, and progress was slow, but within weeks she noticed shifts. The bloating eased first. Then her joints felt a little less stiff in the mornings. She no longer crashed in exhaustion after meals, and for the first time in months she slept through the night.
>
> Sarah still had a way to go. Her genetics carried risk, and she knew there may be harder days ahead. But she also felt something new - hope. By feeding her body in a way it could tolerate and use, she was no longer chasing symptoms. She was beginning to turn the corner.

Phase 6
Live in Rhythm

Length: Ongoing, for life
Pillar Restored: Rhythm

This is not an ending. It's where rhythm becomes your way of life. You'll walk the seasons, work in flow, rest without guilt, and begin to live the way you were always meant to. Present, steady, and fully alive.

Remember the Rhythm

This is the pulse underneath it all.

We weren't made for constant. We were made for pattern. There's a beat in everything, light and dark, rise and rest, hunger and fullness, movement and stillness. You can feel it when the body knows it's time to stop, even if the world keeps going. This is rhythm.

When rhythm is present, the body feels safe. It knows when to open and when to close. It knows when to stretch and when to hold. It doesn't have to guess. It doesn't have to stay on alert. It can land.

But modern life erased the pattern. It stretched the day too long. It blurred the weeks together. It ignored the seasons and flattened the year. And so, the body lost its song.

This section is here to bring it back. You'll remember how to move through time, not just survive it. You'll rebuild your weeks, your work, your rest, your year. Because rhythm is how the body knows where it is. And when it knows where it is, it can come home.

Work in Rhythm

This is where effort becomes aligned.

Something in you was made to build, to shape, to create. To feel the weight of effort, and the deep peace when it's done. But for most, work has become a burden, a drain, a constant climb with no summit. You push through the day, counting hours, watching the clock, and wondering if this is all there is.

But your body knows something else. It remembers a different kind of work, one with pulse, with timing, with purpose and rest woven together. You don't need to quit everything. You just need to adjust how you carry it.

The Function

When work is aligned with rhythm, your nervous system doesn't stay on edge. You cycle through exertion and recovery, instead of staying in constant output.

A good work rhythm charges the system. It builds mitochondrial resilience. It drives focus, creativity, problem-solving. But only when it has boundaries. Work in rhythm lets your brain breathe. It resets your nervous system between effort. It brings clarity instead of fog. It lets your body trust that a pause is coming.

The Fracture

We stopped listening. We ignored the natural cues, like the dip in focus after two hours, or the need to shift tasks when the body starts fidgeting. We filled every space with screens. We blurred the line between work and home. We worked through sickness, through lunch, through weekends. We taught the body that effort never ends, so it stopped recovering.

And now most people live in low-level burnout. Not collapsed. Not thriving. Just ... flat. Like the light's still on, but no one's home.

The Return

- o **Work in 90 - 120 minute blocks, then pause |** Step away, move, and breathe. Let your brain exhale before starting again.
- o **Stop when your body whispers |** Don't wait for it to scream.
- o **Don't fill every break with a screen |** Give your eyes, mind, and body a real pause. Look out the window, enjoy quiet for a moment.
- o **Step outside between tasks |** Even a few minutes of fresh air and natural light can reset your focus.
- o **Create different zones |** Thinking, doing, resting. Give each its own space, even if it's all within the same room.
- o **Batch similar tasks together |** Grouping work stops constant switching and lets your brain stay in one mode for longer.
- o **Use a "bookend" to start and end your day |** A light walk, a stretch, a closing breath. Mark the shift between work and rest.

Signs of Restoration

You start the day steady, not braced. You move through work with focus, not rushed. You notice when it's time to pause, without guilt. You don't crash mid-afternoon or dread the next day. You feel clear, not foggy. Tired, but not depleted. Productive, and still you.

And slowly, you begin to like your work again. Because it no longer owns you. You're sharing the load.

Seasonal Shift

Spring | Seed. Begin. Let energy rise with Spring and use it to start what matters most.

Summer | Do your focused work in the morning, then ease off in the heat. Leave space to celebrate progress and enjoy what's growing.

Autumn | Edit. Refine. Take stock of what's working, and let go of what's not. This is a time for pruning back.

Winter | Step back to strategise and dream. Use the quieter months to rebuild capacity, so you're ready for the next cycle.

Work is not your enemy. Work is not your identity.
Work can be restorative, when it's in rhythm.

Rest in Rhythm

Let the body soften and the system recharge.

Rest isn't doing nothing. It's doing enough, then letting go. It's the space between notes that makes music. But we've forgotten how to stop. Even our rest has become performance. Scheduled, productive, and filled to the brim with "recovery" tasks. We try to rest like we work, with pressure, precision, and guilt.

But true rest is not a checkbox. It's a posture. It's a return. Your body was designed to exhale. To step back. To be quiet. Not just once a year on holiday. But every day. Every week. Every season. You don't need more hours. You need more space inside them.

The Function

Rest resets the circuit. It signals safety to your nervous system. It tells your mitochondria to repair instead of push. When you rest, cortisol drops. Blood sugar stabilises. Digestion improves. Muscles unclench. The brain clears. The breath deepens. Your body exits alert mode, and returns to restore and receive.

But most of all, rest makes room for joy. Because when the system stops bracing, you can actually feel again.

The Fracture

We stopped honouring the pause. We filled every moment with noise. We turned weekends into catch-up days. We blurred the edges of work and home until there were none. And somewhere in the middle, we began to feel guilty for stopping.

We called it laziness. We called it weakness. We forgot that even the earth rests. Even light rests. Even breath rests. We thought we could outpace the need for stillness, but our bodies never agreed. They just got louder.

The Return

- **Just stillness |** Begin with 5 minutes a day. No phone. No plan. Simply sit, breathe, and let your body enjoy the quiet.
- **Sit outside |** Let the sun touch your skin. Feel the breeze. Even a few minutes helps your body remember how to rest.
- **Take small 'gaps' between tasks |** Even a minute of quiet helps reset your focus and gives the body a chance to exhale.
- **End your day with something soft |** Dim the lights, take a warm shower, breathe slow. Small signals like these tell your body it's safe.
- **Once a week, take a deeper pause |** A real rest day. No chores, no catching up. Just space. Let your family see you rest. Let them know slowing down is safe.
- **Protect rest like you protect food or sleep |** It's not a privilege, it's essential. And it's never something to feel guilty about.

Signs of Restoration

You stop rushing even when time is tight. Your breath deepens without trying. You feel soft instead of sharp. You notice light again. Mornings feel less urgent. Even food tastes better. You catch yourself smiling, for no reason at all. You're no longer running from rest. You're receiving it.

Seasonal Shift

Spring | Energy rises, but rest is still needed. Take breathers between fresh starts so you don't burn out before things have even begun.

Summer | Rest in the heat. Find shade, drink water, move softly. Balance the long days with small pauses.

Autumn | Begin to pull back. Let go of what's not needed. Let your weekends slow. Give yourself space to settle into a slower rhythm.

Winter | Deep rest. Lean into early nights and quieter days. Do less, without guilt. This is the season for repair.

Rest isn't falling behind. Rest is wise.

Play in Rhythm

Let life spark and watch joy return.

Play is not just for children. It's for anyone with breath in their lungs and fire still flickering in their chest. You were made to move freely. To laugh unexpectedly. To create something that doesn't need to be useful.

But most people have forgotten how. They've grown serious, efficient, burdened. Somewhere along the way, play got labelled as childish, unproductive, or selfish.

But your body remembers. It remembers the charge that comes when you dance, when you make something with your hands, when you sing off-key, when you chase a ball, or a dog, or a dream. Play is not wasted time. It's joy.

The Function

Play resets the nervous system. It switches the brain from defence to creativity. It clears cortisol. It boosts oxytocin. It opens the breath. Play reminds your system: "I am safe". And safety is what lets you heal.

The Fracture

We outgrew play, or so we thought. We told ourselves to "get serious." We filled our time with goals and obligations. We swapped wonder for worry. And even our hobbies started to look like work.

We forgot how to be unproductive on purpose. We forgot how to be silly. We forgot how to be light. And the body, began to brace.

The Return

You don't need to be good at it. You don't need to schedule it. This isn't about adding something. It's about remembering something. Try:

- **Dance to one song a day** | Alone. Silly.
- **Sing** | Off-key. Loudly.
- **Doodle** | Even badly.
- **Laugh with a friend** | Be around people who make you happy.
- **Wear something playful** | A colour, a texture, something that makes you smile.
- **Make something by hand** | A scarf, a bracelet, a garden bed.
- **Watch something that makes you laugh** | Really laugh.
- **Let your body move** | Like it used to as a kid, on the beach, in the rain.
- **Say yes to spontaneity** | Chase the dog. Climb the rock. Splash the puddle. Let small, unexpected moments turn to joy.

Signs of Restoration

You feel lighter, even if nothing has changed. You laugh without planning to. You feel the charge come back to your system. Your face softens. You wake up with ideas instead of dread. You feel alive again. And not because everything's fixed, but because something in you has reawakened.

Seasonal Shift

Spring | Try something new. Let curiosity lead. Take a class, explore a trail, plant something. Small fresh starts wake up joy.

Summer | Be outside. Move, swim, laugh, share meals with friends. Let long evenings stretch out with stories and simple fun.

Autumn | Slow down and gather. Turn what you've grown into joy - a meal, a painting, a song. Let it make you smile.

Winter | Lean into cozy joy. Games around the table, firelight, and shared meals. Let comfort and friendship carry you through the Winter.

Play isn't a distraction.
It's a return. To joy. To you.

Walk the Seasons

This is where time curves back into rhythm.

Most people don't know what season their body is in, they just keep going. Same routine, same food, same pace, all year. But your body knows. Not by the calendar, but by light. The amount of daylight, the angle of the sun, the feel of the morning air. These are cues your body still listens for, even if your schedule doesn't.

We weren't made to live the same way every month. We were made to move with the year. To shift. To arc. To return. Each season brings a different signal to your nervous system. Each solstice and equinox marks a turning.

You don't need to follow them perfectly. You just need to notice. When you start to live with the seasons, you begin to feel held again. Like the year itself is a rhythm your body can trust.

The Four Turns of the Year

These four turning points are not abstract, they are light-based. They mark real, visible shifts in the environment and in your body's biology. They also signal the true beginning of each season, not by date, but by light. When you notice them, you reconnect with the cycle your body runs on.

1. Spring Equinox | The Reawakening

Equal light and dark

The light returns in balance. Day and night stand even, and your body feels it. This is the gentle rise. Not a sprint. A stirring. The cold begins to lift. The mornings stretch longer. Your body starts to crave movement, air, nature, and light. It's time to begin again, slowly. Clear space. Let breath lead. Wake gently from Winter's depth. This is emergence. Trust the slow rise.

2. Summer Solstice | The Peak

Fullest light

The light is full now. Long days. Short nights. This is the body's natural high tide. Energy wants to move outward, toward work, expression, doing. You feel more charged. This is not a season of stillness. It's a season of energy. Let your mornings hold movement. Let your evenings be cool. Let meals be lighter, fresher. You're not meant to hold this peak forever. Use what's needed. Let energy flow through.

3. Autumn Equinox | The Pull Inward

Equal light and dark again

Light and dark meet again, but now the light is falling. The days shorten. The air changes. The body starts to slow. You feel it in your pace. In your breath. It's a season of finishing, not beginning. Let what's done be done. Cut the noise. Clear the clutter. This is not a collapse, it's a clearing. Health is not always built by adding. Sometimes it's built by release.

4. Winter Solstice | The Resting

Fullest dark

The darkest point. The deepest pause. But not the end, the root. You are still alive here. Just slower. Deeper. This is where the body resets. More sleep. More stillness. Heavier food. Less output. Don't push. Don't launch. Don't demand energy that isn't ready. Let the dark be honoured, not in words, but in rest. You are not broken. You are wintering. And beneath the stillness, strength is forming.

The Function

Most people think they're tired or broken. But often, they're just out of rhythm with the year. Trying to run in Winter. Trying to launch in Autumn. Trying to reset in Summer. Trying to reflect in Spring.

When you return to the seasonal pulse, you don't need to force health. It emerges. You'll crave different foods. You'll shift your routines. You'll make space when it's time to make space, and you'll rise when it's time to rise. This isn't a casual belief. It's biology. Your body was designed to shift with the year.

The Return

Start by simply noticing the light. Ask yourself: what time does the sun rise now? How does the morning feel on your skin? What colour does the sky take on in the evening around six o'clock? And how is your body responding to these changes? The answers will shift week by week, and month by month.

Once you begin to notice, you can start to move with it. Let the change in light shape your rhythm. When mornings grow earlier, rise with them. When evenings draw in, let your body wind down sooner. As the light changes, so can the way you eat, the way you move, even the way you work can change.

This isn't about strict schedules. It's about letting the seasons take the lead again. Instead of fighting against the natural flow of light, begin to follow it. Step by step, your body remembers how to move in time with the world outside, and life begins to feel steadier, clearer, and more alive.

The seasons are not tasks. They are reminders.
That everything in nature pulses, and your body is no different.

Phase 6 | Rhythm Checklist

This phase is about living in rhythm - light and dark, work and rest, effort and ease. Keep it simple, enjoyable and you. This is your rhythm.

Work

- ☐ Work in 90 - 120 min focus blocks. Step outside between blocks.
- ☐ Pause when the body whispers - don't wait for it to yell.
- ☐ Protect a real lunch break away from the desk.

Rest

- ☐ Take 5 minutes daily with no phone or plan - just stillness.
- ☐ Evening downshift - shower, breath reset, or gentle stretch.
- ☐ Have one full rest day each week - no catching up, no guilt, just rest.

Play

- ☐ Daily spark - one song danced, one laugh shared.
- ☐ Say yes to one spontaneous moment each week.
- ☐ Make something by hand - no pressure, just for fun.
- ☐ One undistracted conversation daily.

Seasons

- ☐ At the four turns, review and adjust sleep, meals, movement, light.
- ☐ Spring - Begin gently, start new, but don't start everything at once.
- ☐ Summer - Do focus work early, evenings light and social.
- ☐ Autumn - Edit, finish, and let go. Simplify.
- ☐ Winter - Deepen sleep, shorter days, slower training.

Phase 6 | A Day in Rhythm

Morning

At sunrise, set your water in the light. Step outside barefoot, grounding as you stretch while the sun rises. When you return, drink mineral-rich, structured water. A habit that carries through your day.

Sit to a hearty breakfast. High-fat, animal-based food, cooked with intention. Afterwards, electrolytes help steady and charge your body.

If there is time, you head to the ocean. A short session of bodyweight strength afterward warms you. Red light follows, supporting recovery and reminding your body it can heal.

Then work begins. Not rushed, not blurred. You carry it in blocks, with pauses between. You step outside, let the light touch your skin, let your mind reset. Work has a pulse now. Effort, then release.

Midday

Pause to meet the sun. You stay a little longer these days. Then loosen your body with a short stretch before sitting down to a full but simple lunch. Lamb or beef with butter folded in. Steady food for the afternoon. No rush. No snacks. Just real fuel.

Work continues, but with rest. A walk, a few breaths with eyes closed, or a moment of stillness. Small pauses hold the work steady.

Evening

Dinner comes early and light, though some nights the body is still satisfied. After eating, take electrolytes, then walk at sunset, barefoot, watching the light fade.

As the house grows quiet, there is space for play. A song, a laugh, a stretch, a silly moment that loosens the edges of the day. Then you read, you talk, you rest.

When sleep comes, the bedroom is cool and dark, layered with natural fibres. In bed, five minutes of gentle breathing settles you. Sleep comes not by force, but because your body trusts the rhythm now.

Seasons

And beneath it all, the year carries you. In Spring, your mornings stretch longer, meals grow lighter, your body craves movement. In Summer, you rise earlier, work in the morning, rest in the heat. In Autumn, you slow, clear, refine. And in Winter, you give yourself the deepest pause. More sleep, heavier food, less demand. You no longer fight the seasons. You walk with them. You let them teach you when to build, when to burn, when to rest, and when to rise again.

A Life in Rhythm | Amber's Seasons

Amber is 29, surrounded by friends and successful in her career, but quietly she felt flat. Life seemed heavier for her than for those around her. She tried hard. Pushing through work, chasing goals, getting into shape. But every Summer, when her friends were most active, she collapsed. No matter what she did, it felt like she was always out of step. She was exhausted, and burned out from pushing when her body wanted to rest. Amber's rhythm was upside down.

She began experimenting with a new approach - honouring the seasons instead of fighting them. She allowed Winter to be quieter, leaning into warmth, sleep, and deeper rest. In Spring, she lightened her meals, moved more freely, and noticed her body shedding weight without the strain she once felt. Summer became a time of expression, energy, and connection - when she could play, create, and shine without running on empty. Autumn brought a chance to tidy, simplify, and let go.

It took time, but Amber began to feel her spark return. Her hormones steadied, her sleep deepened, and she no longer felt like she was dragging her body uphill all year round. She wasn't just working less - she was working in time. By listening to the seasons, she found she could finally move through life with a sense of ease.

The Final
Word

What Comes Next?

You've made it through. That matters. Many begin but don't finish, but you did. Pause here for a moment and let yourself see it. You walked with it. That's no small thing.

Yet this is not the end. It's the beginning. Rhythm is not something you master once and then never lose. It is lived, lost, and found again. Each time you return, it grows steadier in you. So do not regret the days you forget. They are not failure. They are the doorway back. And when you fall away, because you will, because you are human, come back gently. One breath. One step outside in the light. One meal eaten slowly. One night where you let the dark hold you. These are the anchors. Small. Steady. Strong.

Now, as you stand at the end of this path, look back. Were there pages you skimmed past? Sections that felt heavy, or that you weren't ready for? Go there again, but with new eyes. With the body you've been tending. With the rhythm you've begun to restore. You may notice something you missed, or feel something that wasn't possible the first time. And if not, that's fine too. This way isn't a sprint. It's a spiral.

Remember, this is a map. Keep it close. Let it travel with you. Reread a chapter five times if you need to. You'll notice different things each time, because you'll be different each time. Health isn't about knowing everything. It's about returning, again and again, to what restores.

And know this, what you've remembered here isn't only for you. As you walk it, others will feel it. The steadiness in your breath will steady them. The rhythm in your days will remind them of their own. You don't need to explain it. Your living will speak louder than words.

So take what you've found here and carry it forward. Into your own body. Into your home. Into the lives you touch. Let rhythm ripple outward, quiet but sure.

This isn't the end. It's the beginning. Now walk it, and let others see the way.

You've walked this far,
and something in you has shifted.
You've touched rhythm again.
You've felt it in your breath, in the quiet,
in the warmth rising inside.

Let the rhythm be your guide now,
not mine, not another's,
but the one your body remembers.

Finishing Up
Appendix

Reference Map

This table shows the seven layers of the body's circuit, the pillars that support each one, and the phases that help bring it back into flow. You can see the overlap between layers, and why healing often asks us to tend to many parts of our health at once. The body doesn't work in isolation, and it doesn't heal in isolation.

Circuit Layer	Supporting Pillars	Healing Phases
Reception (Solar Panels)	Light, Rhythm	1, 2, 4, 6
Transmission (Wires)	Water	1
Regulation (Insulation)	Land, Fat	3, 5
Conversion (Engine)	Breath, Light, Water, Fire, Fat, Rhythm	1, 2, 3, 4, 5, 6
Expression (Output Channels)	Breath, Light, Fire, Fat, Rhythm	1, 2, 4, 5, 6
Protection (Shield)	Light, Water, Land	1, 3, 4
Reset (Return Path)	Breath, Light, Land, Rhythm	1, 2, 3, 6

Rhythm Summary

Here's a simple list of the foundations to keep you steady and in rhythm.

Breath

- ☐ Breathe through your nose whenever possible.
- ☐ Practise the Breath Reset daily (4 - 1 - 6 - 1 nasal breathing).
- ☐ Match your breath with gentle movement - walking, stretching.

Water

- ☐ Structure your water with light, swirling and minerals.
- ☐ Drink a glass of water first thing each morning with a pinch of salt.
- ☐ Add an electrolyte mix into your day.

Light

- ☐ Step outside within 30 minutes of waking and watch the sunrise.
- ☐ Get direct outdoor light on your skin. Building tolerance slowly and never burn.
- ☐ Watch the sunset or step outside at dusk to help align your body clock.
- ☐ Dim lights after dark. Use warm lamps and candles to signal evening.
- ☐ Prioritise natural light - use red light therapy devices to fill the gap.

Sleep

- ☐ Avoid caffeine after 2pm to protect sleep.
- ☐ Set a tech-off time (ideally 8pm or earlier).
- ☐ Keep your room dark, cool (16 - 19°C), and free of phones and Wi-Fi.
- ☐ Aim to fall asleep before 10 pm for deepest repair.

Movement

- [ ] Walk outdoors every day, even briefly.
- [ ] Stretch, bounce, or twist the body to keep fascia and joints fluid.
- [ ] Aim for 2 - 3 short strength sessions per week (10 - 20 minutes).

Meals

- [ ] Anchor your first meal to the morning light.
- [ ] Choose heartier meals earlier, lighter meals later.
- [ ] Keep meals within an 8 - 10 hour window.
- [ ] Keep simple fats on hand - tallow, suet, ghee, butter.
- [ ] Buy fresh ruminant cuts that naturally carry fat.
- [ ] Aim for 70 - 85% of calories from fat, 15 - 25% from protein, 0 - 5% from carbs.

Home & Surfaces

- [ ] Open windows daily for 10 - 20 min.
- [ ] Use simple cleaners - vinegar, bicarb, essential oils.
- [ ] Keep dust low with regular cleaning, vacuuming and wiping.
- [ ] Choose natural personal care products.
- [ ] Bare feet on real earth for five minutes daily.

Cold

- [ ] Finish showers cold. Start with 30 seconds, build to 2 minutes.
- [ ] Try a brief ocean dip or cold bath up to the neck.

Rhythm

- ☐ Work in 90 - 120 min focus blocks. Step outside between blocks.
- ☐ Protect a real lunch break away from the desk.
- ☐ Take 5 minutes daily with no phone or plan.
- ☐ Evening downshift - shower, breath, or gentle stretch.
- ☐ Have one full rest day each week.
- ☐ Daily spark - one song danced, one laugh shared.
- ☐ One undistracted conversation daily.
- ☐ At the four seasonal turns, review and adjust sleep, meals, movement, light.

The Return Path

A quiet guide for when life pulls you off rhythm.

Some days, you'll drift. Life will press in, schedules, illness, stress, sleep loss, a snack that turns into a spiral. You might think, "I've lost it. I've undone everything." But that's not how rhythm works. This way of living was never meant to be perfect. It was meant to carry you, even when you wobble. If you've veered off course, here's how to return.

1. Start with Your Breath

Not the plan. Not the food. Not the panic. Just the breath. One full inhale. One soft exhale. This reminds your body, you're still here. Which means you can still return.

2. Find One Anchor

Don't try to fix everything. Just notice. What slipped first? Was it light? Food? Sleep? Stillness? Pick one and begin again there. Often, that one signal will start to pull the others back into place. This isn't a reset. It's a re-anchoring.

3. You're Not Starting from Week 1

You're not starting from scratch. You're starting from experience. Go back to the foundation:
- Get outside and receive light again.
- Drink real, mineral-rich water.
- Eat a grounding, nourishing meal.
- Stretch.

- Go to bed at the right time.

In just a few days, your system will begin to hum again.

4. Drop the Shame

You didn't fail. Life shifted, and your rhythm flexed. This isn't a punishment. It's a guide back home. Shame keeps you stuck. But rhythm? It flows. It meets you where you are and invites you forward.

5. Remember What This Is Really About

This isn't about perfect habits or clean streaks. It's about real repair. Every time you return, your body learns to trust you again. That trust rebuilds energy, clarity, and peace. You're not just chasing wellness, you're building lasting health.

You're not starting over
You're just coming back. Let that be your rhythm.

If You're Unwell

When sickness hits, don't fight to keep every habit alive. Rest becomes your new rhythm. Keep the simplest anchors you can - gentle light, hydration, warmth, and sleep. As strength returns, layer the others back in one by one. Even recovery can follow rhythm.

When You've Tried Everything | And Still Feel Stuck

An important note on gut overgrowth and biofilm

Sometimes rhythm isn't enough, at least not at first. Sometimes your body is carrying something that doesn't belong. Overgrowth. Fungi. Parasites. Bacteria growing where it shouldn't. You can eat clean, rest well, and drink structured water. And still feel off. Bloated. Tired. Heavy. Lost.

This doesn't mean you're broken. It means the environment inside you has been taken over. And the practitioners who promised to help may not have known how deep it went.

Here's what you need to know. Some organisms hide. They build shields around themselves called *biofilm*. So your body can't see them, and your medicine can't touch them. You may feel like the treatment didn't work. But often, it never reached the target. What can help:

- A comprehensive stool analysis. Not just a guess.
- A practitioner who understands *biofilm*, not just symptoms.
- A protocol that supports your liver and doesn't rush the process.
- Rest between steps. Gentle burn, not a bushfire.
- A willingness to feel worse before you feel better.
- Someone walking with you who listens, not dismisses.

This book doesn't give you that protocol. That's not its role. But this page is here so you don't give up. So you don't think it's in your head. So you don't lose heart. You are not crazy. You are not lazy. You are not too far gone. You may just be dealing with something that hides in layers.

Take this page to someone who listens. Show them what hasn't worked. Ask them what they see. But if they do not see you, if they do not listen to you, walk away. You are worth more than one capsule and a pat on the head. So, keep walking. Until you find someone who listens, who understands, who helps. You are not stuck. You are on the edge of breakthrough.

Troubleshooting & FAQs

Because healing doesn't always move in a straight line.

Your body might respond in ways that feel strange, intense, or unexpected. That doesn't mean you're failing. It means something is adjusting. These moments are invitations to pause and pay attention.

FAQs

"How long will it take?"

There's no single answer. If you've only been unwell for a short while, change can come quickly. But if you've lived with chronic illness for many years, the body often needs more time. A good guide is about a month of steady rhythm for every year you've been unwell. So twenty years of sickness may mean nearly two years of rebuilding. That can feel long, but it's also hope. Every month in rhythm is a layer of repair, a step toward steadiness. Remember, healing isn't linear. Some days you'll feel the shift, other days it will feel quiet or worse. Both are part of the process.

"How do I know it's working?"

You'll notice it quietly, not all at once. Cravings begin to calm. Sleep deepens. Energy steadies. You start to feel more present in your own life, less pulled around by spikes and dips. It may not be dramatic, but the steadiness is the sign.

"Why do I feel worse before I feel better?"

Because your body is clearing and recalibrating. Sometimes healing stirs up what's been stuck. Fatigue, fog, or old symptoms may surface as the system rebalances. It's not always comfortable, but it often means movement is happening underneath. Go gently.

"Is this detox or something serious?"

Detox often comes in waves. You'll feel a shift, then a lull, then another wave. But if symptoms keep worsening or feel alarming, don't push through. Reach out for support. Healing should steady over time, not spiral down.

"Do I have to start over if I mess up?"

No. This isn't a program you can "break." It's a rhythm. You return, that's all. Every return is a reset. Even if you step away for a meal, a week, or a season, you can step back in, and the body remembers.

"I'm not seeing big results. Should I change something?"

Not always. Most people need more light, more salt, more fat, and more rest before anything fancier. These are the quiet foundations that often take longer than we expect. If the base isn't strong, tweaks won't hold.

"How long per phase?"

Four weeks is a minimum, but many people need longer, especially if the body is rebuilding from chronic issues. Let your system, not your calendar, decide when it's ready to move forward.

"Do I have to do cold therapy?"

No, but it helps. Cold wakes the system, supports mitochondria, and resets rhythm. That doesn't have to mean ice baths. Even 30 seconds at the end of a shower, or dipping your face in cool water, teaches your body to adapt. Start where you are.

"Is fasting required?"

No. This is restoration, not restriction. Fast only when you feel strong and steady, never from depletion. In fact, most people need nourishment first. Fasting can come later, when the body is ready, not as a starting point.

"What about methylene blue? I've heard it can support your mitochondria."

Methylene blue has been explored as a way to support mitochondrial energy - especially when used alongside red light therapy.

But these days it's no longer available for general use in many countries and is often prescription-only. If it's meant to come back into your rhythm, it will, through the guidance of a health practitioner.

"I feel upset or emotional."

That's okay. Often the body holds tension until it feels safe, and then it releases through tears, sensation, or emotion. It isn't weakness, it's clearing. Let it flow.

"I'm overwhelmed by all the steps."

You don't need to do it all at once. Let the layers unfold one at a time. Pick one practice, hold it, then add another when it feels natural. Trust your rhythm. Your body already knows the way, your job is to listen.

"I Feel Flat"

If you're doing "everything right" and still feel flat, don't lose heart. It doesn't mean your body is broken, it just means something is still out of balance. Flatness isn't failure, it's your body asking for a closer look.

Often the reason is simple. Sometimes you're not eating enough. Too little food, too little fat, and the body has nothing steady to burn. Sometimes you've tried to detox too quickly, without the minerals to carry it, and the system is left depleted. At other times, it's water and salt out of balance. Too much water without enough salt will leave you heavy, not refreshed.

There can be deeper reasons too. A struggling gallbladder often shows itself in nausea or loose stools after eating fat. Hidden infections, unresolved dental problems, or mould in your environment can keep your immune system switched on, quietly draining energy. Pushing your body through hard training without giving it deep rest will have the same effect. And when your nervous system is locked in alert mode, energy won't flow no matter how perfectly you do everything else.

Feeling flat is the body's way of asking for space. Not more effort, not more rules, but space. Begin by checking the simple things. Enough food. Enough fat. Enough salt. Enough rest. The spark will return.

"I Feel Off"

Symptom	Likely Cause	What to Try
Headache	Detox, tension, dehydration	Hydrate, check - sodium, potassium & magnesium
Light-headed or dizzy	Low salt, overhydration, fasting too long	Sip electrolytes, add unrefined salt, slow fasting
Nausea after eating fat	Gallbladder not ready Low bile	Add lipase, or ox bile, reintroduce fat gradually
Early fatigue	Detox Low fuel	Rest, increase fat, hydrate, allow time to adapt
Lost appetite	Hormone shift	Normal in phases Avoid undereating
Constipation & bloating	Low fat, low salt, gut recalibration	Increase fat, move gently, support with minerals
Cold hands & feet	Under-fuelling Adrenal fatigue	Eat warming foods Increase fat and hydration
Cravings worse	Blood sugar rebalancing	Add more fat, check protein intake, reduce carbs.
Feel "off" but not hungry	Nervous system stuck in "on" mode	Breathe, ground, nourish gently
Slipped up	Guilt loop, overwhelm	You didn't fail. Just return to where you left off.

Oxalate Dumping

If you switched from a high-plant diet and now feel worse (joint pain, skin flare, fatigue, bladder irritation), your body may be clearing stored oxalate. This is called oxalate dumping. It's common during dietary change. Here's what to do:

- **If symptoms flare |** Slow down! Incorporate a small amount of oxalate to slow the dumping, black tea is a common option.
- **Prioritise minerals |** Calcium citrate, magnesium citrate, potassium citrate. They bind to oxalates to help them clear.
- **Epsom-salt foot baths |** Sulphate helps clear oxalate.
- **This will pass |** It often comes and goes in waves. It isn't always pleasant. And it isn't always easy.
- **See Sally Norton's Book |** Toxic Superfoods for more help
- **Support |** There's an excellent Facebook group called "Trying Low Oxalates" should you wish to connect with others.

Choosing a Red Light Device

You don't need the biggest panel or the latest tech. If you're considering red light therapy, here's what to look for:

- **Wavelength |** Choose a device in the 620 - 680nm (red) and 810 - 860nm (near-infrared) range. These are the most studied and biologically effective wavelengths.
- **No flicker |** Flickering light stresses the nervous system. Look for low or no-flicker devices.
- **No heat lamps |** Infrared heat lamps (like saunas) are different. Helpful, but not the same as red light therapy.
- **Check power density |** Look for ~100 mW/cm² at its usable distance. Higher power isn't always better. Too much intensity can overwhelm.
- **Smaller is fine |** A small panel, body wrap, or even a handheld, can still make a difference. Start where you are.
- **Avoid hype |** You don't need add-ons like pulsing, Bluetooth, or colour cycling. You need clean light.
- **Keep your distance |** Keep the panel around 15 - 30cm from the skin (or as recommended in the manual). Too close can deliver too much. Too far may be ineffective.

If you're not sure where to begin:

- Start with natural sunlight.
- Then consider a small device for face, joints, or abdomen.
- Use consistently, not excessively.
- Let your body guide, not marketing.
- You can find more support at www.therhythmofhealth.com.

Bone Broth Recipe

This broth is rich in minerals, amino acids, and collagen. The kind your gut, joints, and skin actually use. It's easy to digest, grounding, and warming. And when it's made fresh, one bowl at a time, it won't trigger histamine responses like store-bought broths can.

Ingredients

- Approx. 500g lamb bones - neck bones or shanks work well
- Filtered water
- Quality salt to taste

Method

- Boil bones for 5 minutes, then pour out the water. This quick boil removes residue and lowers histamine risk.
- Refill the pot with fresh filtered water, just enough to cover.
- Add quality salt.
- Bring to a gentle simmer.
    - *Histamine-friendly:* Let it cook for 60 minutes. Lid *off.*
    - *If histamine isn't an issue:* Let it cook for up to 12 hours. Lid *on.*
- Check regularly. You may need to top up the water slightly, but allow it to reduce so the broth becomes rich and flavoursome.
- Taste and add more salt if needed.
- Strain and drink slowly. Don't rush it. Let your body receive it.

If You Want to Go Deeper

Some people will feel ready to keep learning after they finish. There are plenty of books, podcasts, and online groups out there. Some can bring useful context, language, or clarity. Others may confuse or distract. You don't need to agree with every word you come across. Notice what resonates, leave what doesn't, and go gently. Let your body guide what you take in.

Further Support

If you'd like to keep walking this path, I'll be building resources and practical help on my website over time. There may be tools, guides, or simple next steps to make the rhythm easier to live day by day. It's not another program, just a place to keep exploring if you want to. You can visit: **www.therhythmofhealth.com**

You were never broken

Only out of rhythm

Now the rhythm is yours again

www.ingramcontent.com/pod-product-compliance
Lightning Source LLC
Chambersburg PA
CBHW031147020426
42333CB00013B/544